MORE
MOVING
EXPERIENCES

MORE MOVING EXPERIENCES

Connecting Arts, Feelings, and Imagination

Teresa Benzwie

Illustrated by Robert Bender

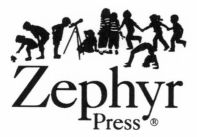

Zephyr Press ®

REACHING THEIR HIGHEST POTENTIAL

Tucson, Arizona

More Moving Experiences
Connecting the Arts, Feelings, and Imagination

All ages.

© 1996 by Zephyr Press

Printed in the United States of America

ISBN 1-56976-032-2

Editors: Stacey Lynn and Stacey Shropshire
Illustrations: Robert Bender
Cover: Robert Bender
Design and production: Daniel Miedaner

Zephyr Press
P.O. Box 66006
Tucson, Arizona 85728-6006

Library of Congress Cataloging-in-Publication Data are available.

DEDICATION

To my family who means the world to me
Lawrence Kirk Bender
Craig Samuel Bender
and Robert Bender

My three fabulously creative beautiful sons who are following their own
individual paths and who are always inspiring me.

To my daughters-in-law
Charmaine Bender
and
Christine Bender
who have enhanced my life with their love and imagination

and to my darling granddaughter
Briana Renée Bender
whose life is full of imagination and sweetness

CONTENTS

Forewords   viii

Acknowledgments   x

Introduction   xii

Peace

One World   2

The Beautiful You   15

Dancing the Web   18

Understanding Differences   23

Transitions

Mother's Day and Father's Day   39

The Egg and the Chicken   51

Caterpillars and Butterflies   54

A Tree Surviving in a Crowded Forest   58

Opposites

Near and Far   65

Over and Under   71

Negative and Positive   78

On and Off   79

Large and Small   85

Fast and Slow   88

Wide and Narrow   90

Push and Pull   96

Tight and Loose   103

Up and Down, High and Low, or Rise and Sink   104

Ending and Beginning   109

Light and Heavy   110

Strong and Gentle   113

In and Out   114

Catching and Letting Go   120

Open—Closed   122

Acknowledging

Expressing Feelings 130

Clay and Play 133

Scarves 134

My Hero 136

Bouncing Names 138

Names and Feelings 140

Magician 141

Learning about Me 142

Self-Awareness, Other Awareness 144

Body Collage 148

Hands and Feet 151

Shadows 152

Games

Games 154

    Pass the Shoe 154

    Car Wash 155

    Commands and Obedience 155

    Cradle Pass 156

Trusting Improvisation 157

    Blind Walk 157

    Circle of Friends 158

    Jelly Roll 159

    Rocking 160

    Tinickling 160

More Curriculum Areas

Wind and Leaves 162

Circles 165

Clocks 175

Animals 179

Suggested Art Materials 181

Appendix A: Movement for the Older Adult 183

Appendix B: Movement Specialist 191

Appendix C: Movement Workshop 201

Professional Organizations 203

Suggested Readings 205

FOREWORD

by Susan W. Stinson

When I first met Teresa Benzwie at a conference on movement and learning for young children, she struck me as one of the most authentic, open, positive, and loving people I had ever met. She also had incredible clarity of vision, recognizing that shared creative movement experiences can be a way to help all ages of people discover (and love) the world, one another, and themselves.

Over the years, I have recognized that these first impressions were not misleading. I have also come to respect the basis out of which Teresa's work comes. Her twenty-five years of teaching inner-city children in New York and New Jersey, leading workshops with adults and children, sharing her ideas with colleagues, and most recently working as a dance therapist have given her a wealth of experience. The activities she suggests in her books are ones she has tried herself in multiple settings.

For Teresa, learning, moving, and imagining are all-of-a-piece, and the world is a place of multiple connections. She knows that the affective, cognitive, and psychomotor dimensions of a person are thoroughly interconnected: learning involves active participation; both learning and doing require a positive sense of self and further contribute to it.

This latest work, as well as Dr. Benzwie's others, gives a glimpse of the remarkable spirit of Teresa Benzwie, as she shares herself so honestly on page after page. Teachers, therapists, parents, and other caregivers are sure to find ideas they will use and be touched by the life-affirming presence of this generous author.

Susan W. Stinson, Ed.D.
Department head and professor of dance
University of North Carolina at Greensboro

FOREWORD

by Sarah Hilsendager

More Moving Experiences: Connecting the Arts, Feelings and Imagination reaches into the very essence of dance and dance making as life experience. This creatively conceived, richly illustrated book shares with the reader the sparkle, the energy, and the animation that is the foundation of Dr. Benzwie's approach to sharing with children through the medium of movement. In her unique way, the author blends knowledge and understanding gained through years of practical classroom experience with imaginative and insightful ideas, strategies and applications that can be used in a wide variety of creative movement settings. *More Moving Experiences* touches the dancer in us all, because it stimulates our own imaginations, explores our personal sources and feelings of and through movement, and encourages us to embrace the arts as an inherent part of our daily lives. We are invited to enter the world of active engagement and invention, releasing ourselves to the wonderment and fascination of creative exploration.

I highly recommend this book to anyone who cares about children, about their growth as creative human beings, and about the worlds of interaction that are opened and extended through the arts.

Thank you, Teresa, for sharing your magic—its contribution knows no bounds.

Sarah Hilsendager, Ed.D.
Professor and Chairperson, Dance Department
Temple University

ACKNOWLEDGMENTS

There are many people I have been grateful to in the last few years as I have been writing this book. *More Moving Experiences* really belongs to all of you who have inspired me through your love, generosity of time, talents and participation in the arts.

Special thanks go to my son Robert Bender, who again allowed my ideas to come alive through his marvelous illustrations. Your generous contributions of time and brilliance brought life and energy to the creative movement experiences, allowing the children to dance right off the pages. Thank you so much, Robert. I feel so proud and lucky to have been able to collaborate with you once again.

I drew upon Louise Kelsey's expertise in the special classroom to expand my ideas for this population. Working with Louise showed me how children with special needs can be partially or completely included in the regular classroom. Louise added many ideas contributing to special needs. Thank you, Louise, for helping to make this book so much richer and expanding *More Moving Experiences* to reach special needs populations.

Thank you, Joey Tanner, for believing in my work and encouraging me to write *More Moving Experiences.* Without your loving motivation this book would not have happened. Special thanks also goes to Stacey Lynn and Janie Brewster, who were my advocates and editors and who sustained me through the process.

Thank you, Tracy Miller and the Board of Education of the Cherry Hill schools for allowing Robert Bender and me to come into your schools to work with your children.

I am particularly grateful to Ron Roberts and Adrean Hill, who allowed Robert and me to come into their physical education classes over a three-year period to use the movement experiences with their classes. Thank you so much, Ron and Adrean, for your kindnesses and support.

Thank you also to the spirited and cooperative children from Ron and Adrean's physical education classes at Kingston, Thomas Paine and Russell Knight schools, during the years 1991 to 1994. Your willingness to explore these ideas with Robert and me was a joyful and rewarding experience.

Thank you, Christina Bender, my daughter-in-law, for reading through the manuscript with your artistic eye and offering some zany additions.

Thank you, Charmaine Bender, my daughter-in-law, for all your helpful ideas. I enjoyed watching my granddaughter Briana while you tucked yourself away to edit.

Thank you, Diane Belden, for trying out some of these ideas with your four-year-old son, Michael, and sharing his reactions and thoughts with me. You both were very helpful.

Upon perusing my manuscript on her holiday weekend, Sheela Peace spontaneously chose to give up her vacation time to edit. Thank you, Sheela. I am grateful for your knowledge and support.

Many other friends and students took the time to read through the manuscript to help in the editing process. Thank you, Sheila Greenberg, Harlene Galen, Barbara Kahn, Deborah Curtiss, Katherine Galiszuski, Mary Ellen Ganey and Anita Mizrachi.

Thank you also to my students from the spring 1994 class in therapeutic applications of dance in education at Hahnemann University Department of Mental Health Sciences: Claudia Eng, Leigh Gellman, Dawn Morningstar, Nancy Crafts and Mary DeArnent. Your comments were helpful.

Thank you, JoAnn White, for collaborating with me on dance for the older adult. Your input was extremely productive and useful.

Many thanks to Rosanne Regan Hansel, director of the Gloria Dei Preschool, for allowing me to participate and work with the preschool children and their "huggers" (older adults).

Thank you to Randy Olmstead of Chime Time, who donated some of the equipment to be used in the classes illustrated within. Thank you for the Body Sox, Co-Oper Band and Parachute. The materials were extremely helpful and enjoyable to use.

Special thanks and love to Albert Benzwie whose creative spirit lives on.

Many thanks for the outstanding skills and energies of Zephyr Press. You all are deeply appreciated.

To all of you, my gratitude and appreciation for helping make *More Moving Experiences* a reality.

Teresa Benzwie

INTRODUCTION

Fantasy

Sometimes we hear adults say that some children and adolescents have their heads in the clouds, can't face reality or are always in a fantasy world, as if this state were undesirable. I honor and appreciate the imaginative, creative, fantasy world as a bridge to fulfilling wishes. Learning is such an inward journey, building on a collection of mutually enriching experiences. The more we can facilitate this idea of learning, the more we connect our children to themselves, one another, and their world. Learning and personal growth are an active collaboration of unconscious and conscious feelings and thoughts dealing with the journey of the client or student.

One has to imagine before new ideas and ways of doing things can be created. Many of the inventions we take for granted and use in our daily lives were first fantasies. So I encourage all to have dreams and create worlds where you will feel happy and fulfilled. Then you can "come down to earth" to share and live out your fantasies.

The Arts

When I was a child, the arts were my salvation. They enabled me to realize my own potential, empowered me to survive challenges and channel undesirable situations into creative, productive ones.

All of us are artists in that we all have the ability to be creative. Creativity can be expressed in a visual work of art or in mundane tasks. Creativity involves freedom of thought, pushing boundaries, acceptance of and expression of our individuality, risking standing up for our beliefs or changing what is in our power to change. Creativity involves actively taking a part in shaping our lives toward fulfillment and being true to ourselves, our minds, bodies and spirits.

The arts engage students in the art of learning like no other phenomenon. They can flow from one to the other, creating an aesthetic statement as we interact with others in a collage of music, movement and other arts, reflecting our differences while joining together. The arts can validate the child's use of all the senses. They celebrate individuality by helping each child discover his or her expressive potential.

Music can be interpreted in a drawing and art can be interpreted in movement. We can write about what we performed in movement and orally share the whole experience. We can draw our feelings and dance our drawings and accompany each other with rhythm instruments or body sounds. Each time ideas are processed through a different art form, they become deeper, more understandable and expansive.

Movement

Creative movement, the most immediate and accessible of the arts because it involves our own bodies, creates a wonderful self-contained environment conducive to discovery. It is that one powerful, perfect moment fusing time and space in a world of varying tempos. Creative movement releases the flow of energy to our fantasies, feelings and intellect. It can be a powerful tool for change, helping us to become in touch with our bodies, healing our spirits and connecting us to our feelings. Through movement, music, and imagination, it is possible to blend fantasies and realities in a wholeness of being.

We sometimes hear the term "getting back to basics." What can be more basic than our own bodies? We also may hear, "Who, me!? Dance? You must be joking! I never took dance lessons . . . I was always clumsy . . . I have two left feet, I couldn't dance to save my life . . . I'm too fat . . . too short . . . too tall . . . too bony . . . my feet are too big . . ." and so on. The concepts we have of dance and of our own abilities are sometimes misunderstood. Everything we do involves movement. Can you walk across the room? Can you bend down low? Reach high? Can you curl up, stretch out, skip, run, shake your head slowly, turn your arms quickly? Well! You are moving, using your body, feeling your muscles, experiencing your feelings and on your way to dancing.

Funds for supplies are always scarce; working through movement is very inexpensive. All we need are our own bodies, the desire to move and to create a learning environment in which students and teachers may discover together.

Movement as a way of relating helps us enter the child's world, providing an environment to develop unique talents. Children are naturally active learners. We learn a great deal, both consciously and unconsciously, about children through their body language. With the awareness that comes through movement, children's feelings and body expression become one. Children need to come out from behind their desks and use their total selves in their own space to reach their highest potential.

What we accomplish with creative movement might at first seem deceptively simple because, in and of itself, the movements are simple and appear to be obvious. The overall complexity is not apparent until you have worked through the whole range of constantly expanding cognitive abilities, emotional interactions and physical awarenesses. For example, a child's ability to move through space with another person, appropriately responding to the concept of up and down or open and closed, reflects a great deal of control, focus, self-assurance, motor control, understanding of language and ability to control and define personal space.

Although some children do have attention deficit disorder and are hyperactive, others have been misdiagnosed with these problems. They may need to be actively involved through body, mind and feelings, using their natural high energy in the learning process.

The Environment

Creating a supportive, nonjudgmental environment is important in the classroom as well as in the therapeutic setting. Here, children and adults should feel free to make mistakes, to learn from them and explore feelings.

Children constantly give us clues about how they communicate. They are my best teachers because they teach me how they can be reached. We cannot stand outside the experience, but need to be directly involved, taking our cues from the child. All suggestions and ideas are respected as teachers and children together become part of the learning process.

We as parents or teachers do not have all the answers. We can, however, create an environment that will constantly nurture and support the possibility of positive choices that will foster the child's humanity and total growth.

Children with Special Needs

All children, particularly those who have neurological impairment or other physical challenges, need clear messages that they are good human beings and we like and accept them as they are.

Creative movement is a versatile tool for meeting diverse needs. We can adjust movement experiences to accommodate special needs. Contact is required for learning to take place. Movement helps to establish that contact, opening the door for further communication. When a child cannot move her own body, we move it for her. When others are not able to give visual attention, we bring props into their visual field. Ongoing movement experiences seem to help desensitize tactile defensiveness. Bringing children in close proximity to one another through a focus on movement seems to help them become less self-conscious about touching and being touched. Movement experiences enhance and help stimulate all the senses, bringing responses from children who ordinarily have few or none. Such activities may also be used with younger children.

Developing a positive way of relating can help transform acting out behaviors into appropriate positive involvement. Teachers, transforming a negative behavior into a positive productive idea, can help a child feel accepted, important and creatively challenged.

Movement has helped me with many problems with individual children. Sam has a slight case of cerebral palsy and so was cautious when moved. With time and these activities, he became physically and intellectually outgoing. Dawn was very shy and withdrawn. She always whispered and had her arms down at her sides or crossed in front of her. Although she is still quiet, she has become more outgoing in her movements. Michelle, who had brain surgery six weeks before she came to school, constantly needed to hold on to someone for protection. When we were involved in movement, she didn't need to hold on. Given the freedom of movement coupled with warmth and love, many of the children who had physical and emotional trauma in their young lives were able to express their feelings and free their creativity, empowering them to be more intellectually and emotionally whole.

The Process

It is important that activities that begin with teacher and child as partners lead eventually to child and child partnerships and to total group interaction. All children, challenged and able, learn a good deal from one another and need the opportunity to initiate interactions and original ideas. The positive interaction of the group can add strength, with each individual reacting to, adding, receiving and building on the energies of others. The leader, therapist or teacher can facilitate such mutual support and giving.

Humanistic interaction is essential for the growth and positive development of children. Carl Rogers speaks about unconditional positive regard and respect for the needs of each individual and, given a choice, the child will choose what ultimately is good for him or her.

I am often asked what to do with children who do not want to participate. First I must say that no child is ever forced to participate. Some children are afraid to try new things and will stand apart at the beginning of the year just to watch. Eventually, they join in. I often rely on the class's energy and their joyful participation to entice students into eventually participating. Also, I feel there are many ways to participate. For example, if there is a child who is sitting in our circle but not physically involved, I feel she is still participating because she is in our circle. Even if she has her back turned, if she is still in our circle, she is still with us in some way. If she is in another part of the room but watching us, she is participating at some level.

It is a different matter if the child is being disruptive and distracts the group. I will not allow that. I will say it is okay if he doesn't want to do the activity, but I explain that he doesn't have the right to keep the rest of the class from participating. I suggest that he do something quietly to occupy himself. If he goes along with my suggestion, he is respecting what the rest of the class is doing and is participating at a minimal level.

Movement and Age

In movement, there are no age limits and no mistakes. Some of my most interesting ideas come from adult creative movement classes in which a participant misunderstood my directions and created yet another moving experience.

In some of the illustrations, you will see older adults. These people were in "Huggers," a group of older adults who volunteer their time to work with a group of children at Gloria Dei Preschool in Huntington Valley, Pennsylvania. Happily, other preschools across the country are connecting with nursing homes to the benefit of all. Movement is often the bond. The children are validated by the elders and the elders treasure what the children do as well as feeling needed and productive. There is acceptance and nonjudgmental love between young and old. The connection between these two groups is natural as they enjoy the unconditional acceptance and joy that they bring to each other. Here we see how children of all ages, from 3 to 91, can enjoy movement and playing together.

People of all ages can enjoy movement activities, such as mirroring. Although I give only a few examples, you can bring a wealth of your own ideas to integrate movement experiences for young and old.

This Book

Many of the movement experiences I offer go together in a theme. You don't necessarily have to do all of them in the same session, however. Choose one or all as you see fit according to your time restrictions and your students' ability to stay with the experience. You can also decide which activities are age appropriate for your populations and feel free to adjust them accordingly.

Enjoy the learning process, the teaching process and the interaction between your work and children. It can be exciting and enjoyable for both teachers and children. I see creative movement and dance therapy more as a way of relating than as a specific technique. The aim is teaching the children in a way that allows them to give themselves what they need in their lives.

PEACE

Peace begins with ourselves.

When we feel peaceful within,

we feel more peaceful toward one another,

our planet and all its living things.

ONE WORLD

Relaxation

Let's sit in a circle.

We are going to help ourselves feel good.
Make believe one of your hands is giving your opposite arm a bath.
Gently stroke your arm from your shoulder all the way to your fingertips.
Yes, that's good. Softly, gently and slowly.
Stroke your arm lovingly so that it will feel good.
Now do the same using the other hand and arm.

Gently use your fingertips to stroke your face, feeling your nose, eyes, mouth, ears, eyebrows and forehead. Do this lovingly, feeling the shapes.

Now tap gently all over your head as if raindrops were falling on you, tingling and feeling good.

Run your hands down your sides to your legs. Bathe one leg and then the other. Remember to be gentle so that your legs will feel loved.

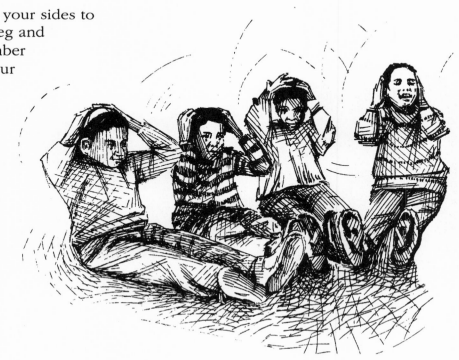

Now let's give our-selves three strokes beginning at the head, down to our shoulders, then sweeping down our sides and finally down our legs.

Ready?
Once, twice,
three times.
Good!

2

Visualization

Breathe in all the pleasurable feelings we created in this room. When we breathe out, we will be breathing out those feelings to others.

S l o w l y   breathing in nurturing feelings.

   S l o w l y   breathing out loving feelings to each other.

   In and *out.*

With every breath we take, we are filling up the entire room with our positive feelings. There are so many positive feelings in this room that they can fill up the whole building. Now everyone in the building can feel our wonderful feelings.

Keep breathing beautiful feelings in and breathing beautiful feelings out. Breathing in and out all the feelings that feel comfortable and warm to you.

Now there are so many pleasant feelings in this building that they are spilling over into the streets and filling up our whole city. The people walking in the street feel them. The people in stores and cars feel them. The cats, dogs, birds and all of the other animals feel our good feelings right at this moment.

Now there are so many delightful feelings filling up this city that they are spilling over the entire state. The fishes in the water feel our good feelings. People working and people playing feel them right now.

There are so many magnificent feelings in our state now that they are spreading to the entire country. Over mountains, through the forests, through the desert, over lakes and rivers everywhere. People throughout our entire country, in their houses or at their jobs, on the street walking or riding, are all feeling wonderful right now. We are spreading beautiful feelings throughout the whole United States.

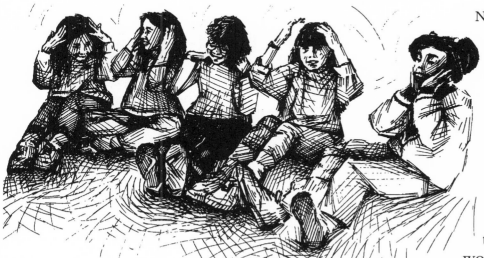

Now there are so many sunny feelings throughout the country that these feelings will be able to cross the oceans to Europe, Asia, Africa and Australia. They will go south to Central and South America and north to Canada. Our terrific feelings are floating throughout the entire world right now. People who are fighting will stop because they feel peaceful. Presidents and heads of state throughout the world are feeling loving and want to have peace. Whales and dolphins are playing, lions and tigers and bears are feeling terrific and the leaf-cutting ants in the rain forest are feeling great. The flowers and trees are feeling bright. All living creatures are feeling glorious right now, because we are sending these feelings to them.

For Children with Special Needs

It may be possible for the children to do "breathing in pleasant feelings" with partners in order to pick up the others' breathing patterns. Partners could be back-to-back or one may lean his or her back against the other's chest. This touching will help children feel each other's rhythm in a nonverbal way.

by Louise Kelsey

Verbal Sharing

How do you feel right now?

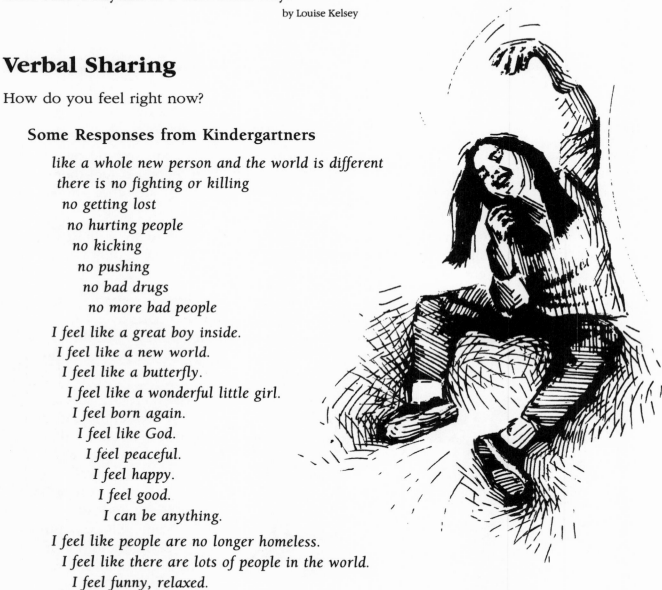

Some Responses from Kindergartners

like a whole new person and the world is different
there is no fighting or killing
no getting lost
no hurting people
no kicking
no pushing
no bad drugs
no more bad people

I feel like a great boy inside.
I feel like a new world.
I feel like a butterfly.
I feel like a wonderful little girl.
I feel born again.
I feel like God.
I feel peaceful.
I feel happy.
I feel good.
I can be anything.

I feel like people are no longer homeless.
I feel like there are lots of people in the world.
I feel funny, relaxed.

Art

Some of you may choose to draw your reactions at this time. Your drawings do not have to look like anything representational. You could create feeling drawings with colors, shapes and designs.

Dancing

Begin to move in your own way with these good feelings. Make it a ***Feeling-Good*** dance.

Begin by s t r e t c h i n g your arms and legs.

Slowly get up to a standing position. Continue your stretching, bending and twisting.

Feel your own healing energy and its goodness.

Move through the space, stretching and reaching, turning and twisting, feeling good.

Do your ***Feeling-Good*** dance.

Let every part of your body feel good dancing throughout all parts of the room.

Be aware of the other dancers so that you don't bump into anyone.

Be generous with the space. Fill it up with your ***Feeling-Good*** dance.

Slowly come to a freeze position, making a sculpture of your feelings.

Look around so that you can see all of the other sculptures and admire them.

Flow Dancing

Without touching, use your hands to trace your body, following its contours and being aware of its shape. Now dance in slow motion toward another person and trace his or her sculpture without touching. Flow freely from one person to another, stopping each time to trace the space around a part of each body. Someone else may be tracing you at the same time. Let this be an ongoing healing dance. Your hands are bringing good energy to others.

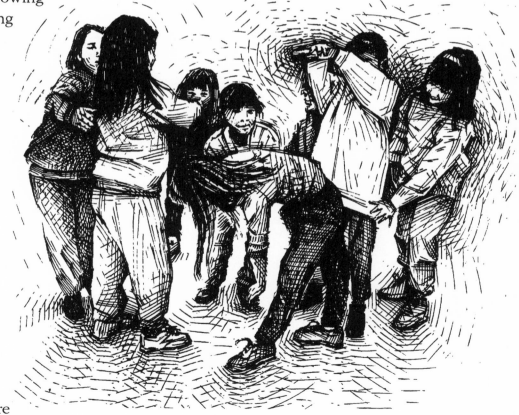

Mirroring

Turning to the nearest person for a partner, do some mirroring. First one and then the other will share her **Feeling-Good** dance. Do it slowly so that your partner can follow you. We all have our own way to feel good, and we will share that way with each other.

Choose another partner to mirror and share your dances.

Change partners as often as time and attention span allow. Peers can often motivate each other with minimal instruction from the teacher.

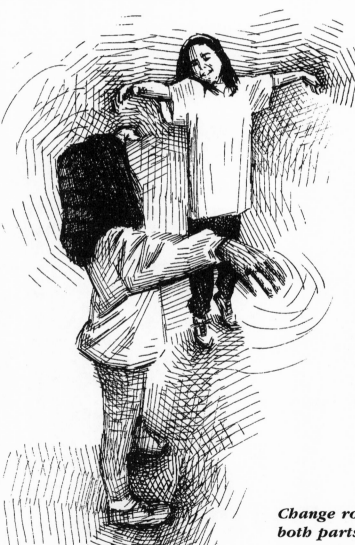

Mirror Variation
Friend/Helper

Work in partners. One person, called the friend, will be in his own world, not paying attention to his partner. The other, whom we will call the helper, is going to try to enter that world by mirroring her friend's movements. Try to respect the friend's space while you position yourself near him. Try to get your friend's attention by entering his world through mirroring. Be sensitive to how close your friend will let you get. Mirror all his movements and body positions, as subtle as they may be. Friend, you will be aware of your helper trying to make contact with you and also be aware of your feelings while she is doing so. When you are ready you may let your helper into your world. Helper, be aware of your feelings as you try to make contact. Be aware of your frustration or satisfaction as you work.

Change roles so that each may experience both parts.

This exercise fosters respect for one another by developing sensitivity to body language while trying to establish a relationship.

For Children with Special Needs

An unaffected child can be the mirror and an affected child can be the leader. In this way, the mirror will be able to enter the world of the leader, honoring the feelings and space of the affected child.

Mirrors, as you follow your partners' movements you will be showing your desire to enter their world. Be patient and follow the movements as closely as possible. You are learning a new way of moving. You are expanding your movement vocabulary.

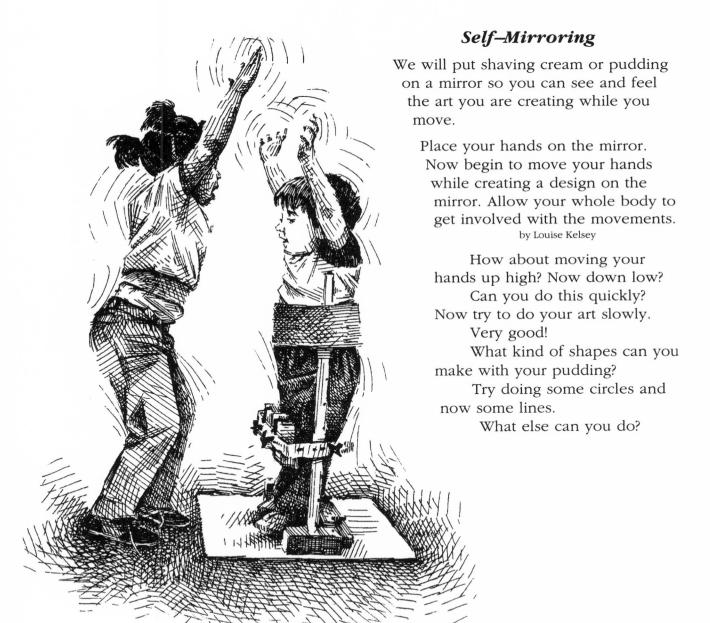

Self–Mirroring

We will put shaving cream or pudding on a mirror so you can see and feel the art you are creating while you move.

Place your hands on the mirror. Now begin to move your hands while creating a design on the mirror. Allow your whole body to get involved with the movements.
by Louise Kelsey

How about moving your hands up high? Now down low?
Can you do this quickly?
Now try to do your art slowly.
Very good!
What kind of shapes can you make with your pudding?
Try doing some circles and now some lines.
What else can you do?

Family Sculpture

Partners, join another pair of partners and become a group of four. This is your family. Create a sculpture by connecting to each other with different parts of your body and on different levels of high, medium and low.

Flow to another level, ending with four different levels, all connected as a family.
Freeze and be aware of where you are in this family.
Again, continue flowing to different levels.
Flow away from your group of four, but not too far. Do your own dance and then come back to your group and connect again.
Leave the group and remember your individual selves.
Create yourself in sculpture form and freeze it. Look around the room at all of the individuals.
Now flow through the space and create a different sculpture that is you.
In slow motion, connect to the nearest person
. . . and release and flow.

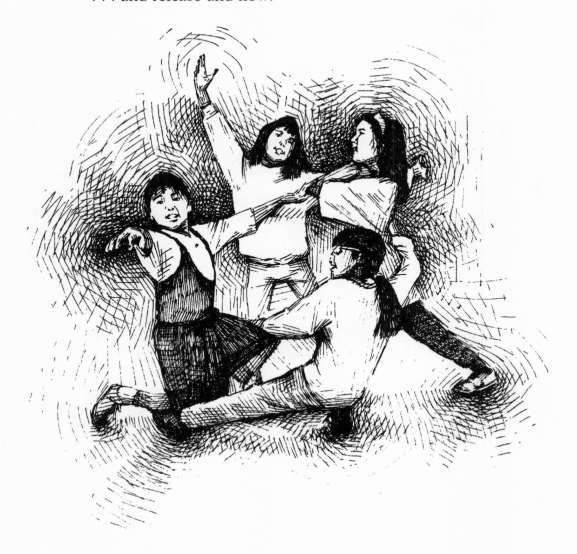

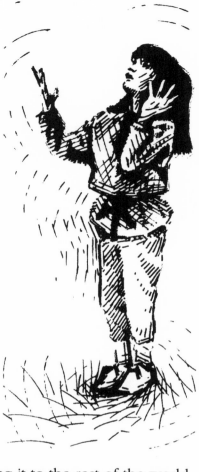

Think to yourself, "Who is this beautiful, unique human being?" and dance the way only you can dance.

Be the special you. Create a sculpture and then connect to another sculpture.

Connect in every way possible with your feet, fingertips, head, with your hips, elbow or shoulder. Connect to as many people as you can.

Now release from them. Take your freedom and create yourself in space.

    Do *your* dance.
        Be who you are and freeze.

In slow motion, connect to the rest of the universe.
    Imagine this whole room is the universe and
        you are one with it.

      Right now connect, and also be yourself.
        Again move through the space.
            Create your genius and explore
                your uniqueness, taking
                this very special
                person who is you
                and again connecting it to the rest of the world.

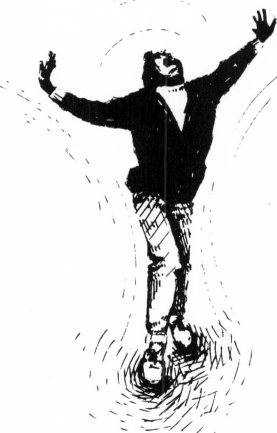

    Connect on as many levels as there are people
        and make one huge sculpture.
           One world.
             Again!

Create that beautiful you.
    Be aware of your body. Stretch it out.
        Make a beautiful shape and feel it.

Feel that beautiful person that is you.
    Feel it and move around this room.
Be it and take this energy, this marvelous energy
    and connect it to the rest of the universe.

Connect on all levels and feel it.
    Feel the energy of the whole universe
        pulsating through your body.
Feel your energy going out and connecting to
    the rest of the world.
Feel it and keep it and flow to a different level
    and connect as one.

Peace Sculpture

Explore moving in a peaceful way throughout the space. Allow your whole body to find different ways to move while experiencing the feeling of peace. Now, one at a time, move into the center of the room and freeze into a peaceful shape. You may want to be low down on the floor, reaching up high, or somewhere in the middle. You may want to attach to some other sculpture person or be separate.

You decide. When everyone is in position, we will have created a peace sculpture.

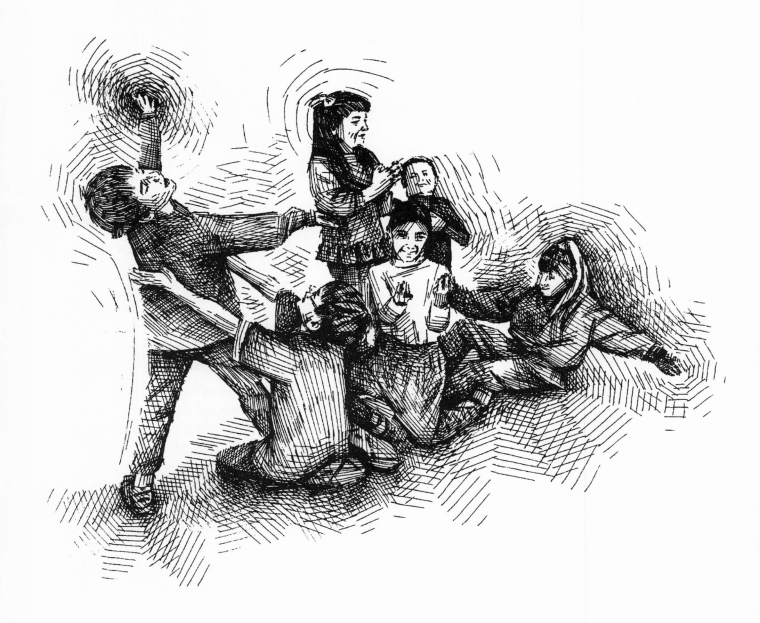

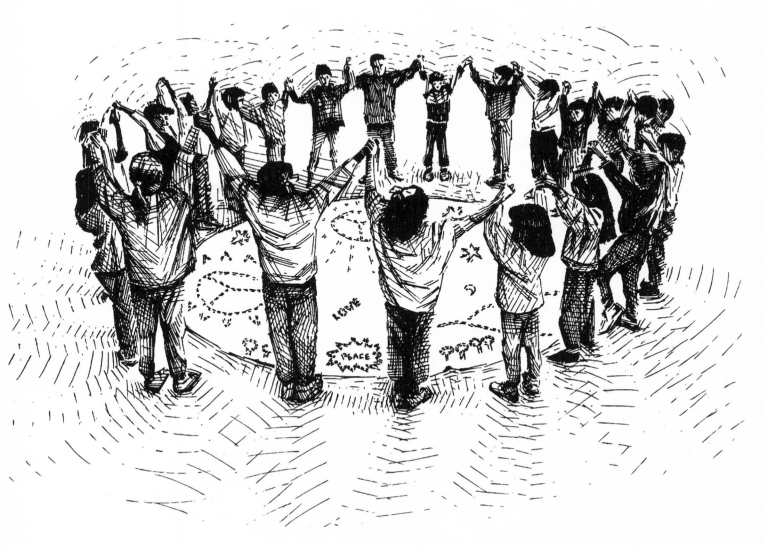

Art

Spread out a huge paper circle, large enough for all of the children to sit around, and give them plenty of markers. I usually use rolled newsprint that I buy by the pound from a newspaper firm.

> Let's sit around this paper circle.
> It is our world.

Take any color you wish and draw or write something about peace. You don't have to stay in one place. You may want to crawl to the center carefully or move around to different spots on the paper. We can fill up the entire world with your drawings and words. Don't forget to write your name. This is your world.

Now that we have finished drawing, let's hold hands and walk around the outside of this circle while we sing "We Are the World. We Are the Children."

Is there another song you would like to sing as we slowly walk around looking at all the beautiful drawings and writings you have made?

Discussion Questions

What would you like to say about this experience?

Would you like to talk about what you drew on our world? How do you feel? How can we help to make our world more peaceful?

What are some things that keep us from having peace?

Can you think of a special time when you felt peaceful? Close your eyes and see that time. What are you doing? Where are you? Is there anyone else with you? What are you wearing? Are you sitting, standing, walking or something else? Picture what you are doing as if it were a movie in your head.

We can open our eyes now and those who would like to may share their experiences.

Close your eyes again and this time see if you can think of a time when you felt like fighting or really did fight. What was that like? Open your eyes now and if any of you would like to share your experience, we would like to hear it.

What were the consequences of your fight?

Did your fight solve the problem?
How do you feel when you see others fight?

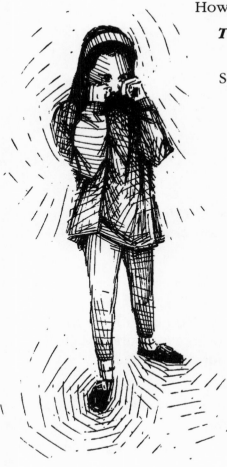

This may open the discussion regarding parental fights.

Some responses relating to fights were

> I felt scared.
> I felt upset.
> I felt angry.

Hanging our Peace Mural

Where can we hang our peace mural? We can put it up in our classroom or in the lobby of our school.

Maybe we can put it up in the library or even send it to the president of our United States.

Do you have any other ideas of where we could put our peace mural?

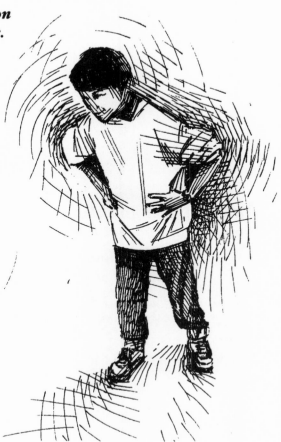

Game

Tape a square to the floor large enough for ten children or the number you are working with to squeeze into with some difficulty.

I would like all of you to fit within this small square on the floor. No part of your body may touch the floor outside this square. As a group you have to figure out how you are going to achieve this. See how you can work together.

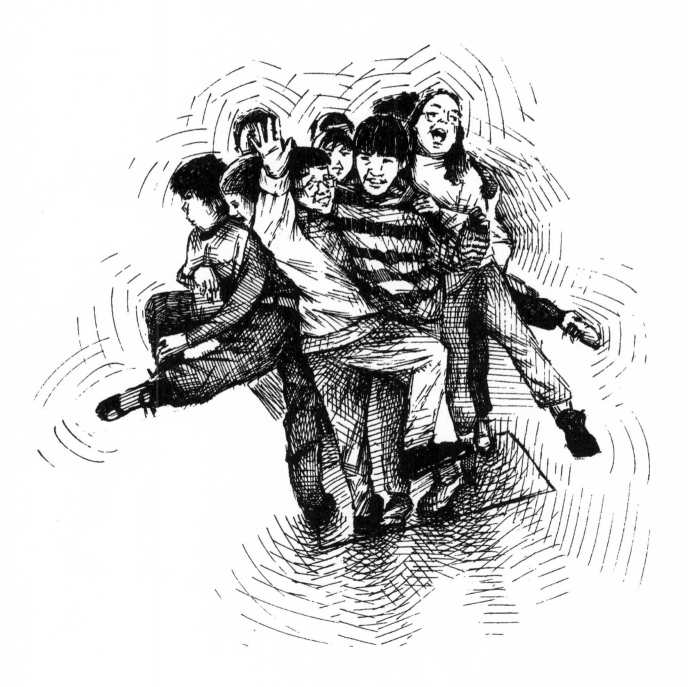

For Children with Special Needs

Although these activities came out of experiences in a special needs classroom, all children may enjoy them at an appropriate age.

In one of my classes a child with pervasive developmental disorder was tapping his wrist with his other hand in self-stimulatory behavior. We brought this child into the group experience by giving him a partner to tap his wrist for him with a small ball.

Tap your partner's wrist with the small soft ball. *Tap, tap, tap* with the ball. *Tap, tap, tap* the ball on Megan's wrist. Repeat this phrase over and over again.

What other parts of your partner's body can we tap with the ball? *Tap, tap, tap* with the ball. *Tap, tap, tap* the ball on Megan's hand. Sing this phrase in rhythm the same way, over and over again.

What other part of your partner's body can we tap with the ball?
Tap, tap, tap with the ball. *Tap, tap, tap* the ball on Megan's knee.

Extending the activity to other parts of the body promotes generalization of concepts and introduces the same idea in different ways facilitating divergent thinking.

Can you feel that rhythm?
Is your partner looking at you now?
Do you want to be closer to your partner?
If you do, ask for permission to get closer.
Does it feel good to connect?

These activities help build bridges connecting the rhythms of the inner and outer world of the child.

Try this with balls of different textures, weights and sizes. You could use soft sponge balls, yarn balls, or hard rubber knobby balls.

Singing the same line over and over increases awareness and helps focus attention.

Mitts
by Louise Kelsey

Some children with special needs can receive more sensory feedback if they stroke themselves using hand mitts with different textures.

Body Cream
by Louise Kelsey

Rubbing on body cream is another way for children to receive tactile stimulation. They can do this themselves or for each other to promote socialization.

THE BEAUTIFUL YOU

Dressing Up

Do you know the beautiful you?
Do you know the handsome you?

Find some scarves and pieces of fabric, and color yourself beautiful.
Oh, how beautiful and handsome you are!

Look at all the colors and costumes you are creating.
Everyone is so magnificent. Together we can make a rainbow.

One four-year-old boy, Michael, thought the fabrics were "girl things" and so we added men's ties to the collection. He then chose to use the scarves.

Walking Down the Runway

One at a time, you may walk down the runway as the most beautiful person in the whole world. Everyone will clap for you.

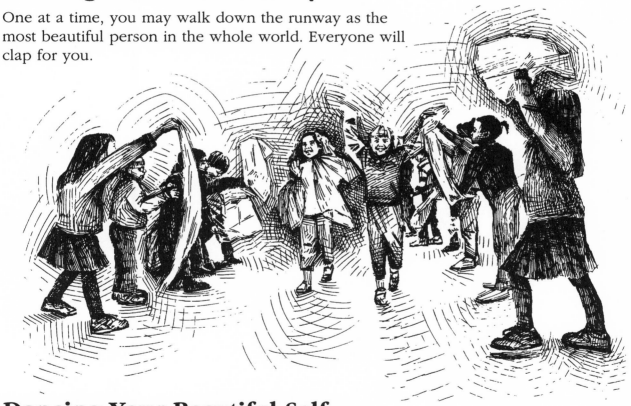

Dancing Your Beautiful Self

Do your beautiful dance, flowing gracefully, dancing the beautiful you as you move.

Videotape

This might be a good opportunity to videotape the children, giving them feedback on their beautiful selves and providing a way to get in touch with their positive self-image.

Names with Positive Affirmations

Let's stand in a circle.

One at a time you will enter the center of the circle and say your name with a word that wonderfully describes you.

For example, "I am talented Liz."

Everyone say, "She is talented Liz."

We will say it over and over as Liz expresses these words in a dance.

Now Liz will come back into the circle and the next person will go into the center of the circle and say his name.

Let's use two words to describe you.

"Hello, I am brilliant, courageous Albert."

Everybody may say, "He is brilliant, courageous Albert."

We will go around in the circle until everyone has a chance to say their name with a positive word and receive reinforcement from the group.

You can also do this exercise using words that begin with the first letter of your name such as, "I am Sensitive Sandra."

Photographs

We will take a photograph of how you feel at this moment and place it around the room so that it will provide a permanent image of your unique self-expression. Give me a word that describes that feeling and we will write it under your photograph.

Use a Polaroid camera. The children will eventually take home these photographs.

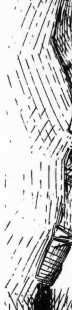

Dancing Your Name

Choose three words that describe you.
Now dance these words as you say them, using your whole body.

Briana is intelligent
    kindhearted
        and beautiful.
Emerson is handsome
    generous
        and loving.
           Say it again and again.

Partners

Sit down facing your partner with your eyes closed.
I would like you to see yourself as a new person discovering the world for the first time.

Visualize a flower.   Describe it to yourself.
Visualize a cloud.   Describe it to yourself.
Visualize the grass.   Describe it to yourself.
Visualize the sun and how it feels.

Visualize a warm bath and imagine how that feels.
When I ask you to open your eyes, you will see your partner
as if for the first time.
The nicest, prettiest or most handsome person you ever saw.
You will see your partner as if you were an artist.
See the shapes, colors, lines and planes of his or her face.
See the beauty shining from within.
Open your eyes now.
Look at your partner in total silence.
No judgments and no labeling.
Really see her or him. See the beauty shining from within.
Now you may share your feelings with your partner.

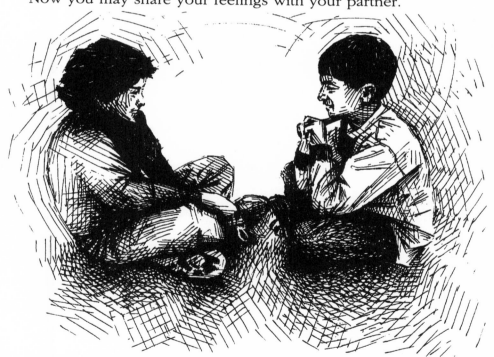

Take a few minutes to tell your partner about all of his or her positive qualities.
Now you may pick one that you think represents yourself best.

Let's walk through the room, saying your name and the one word you chose to as many
people as possible.

DANCING THE WEB

Body Awareness

Let yourself be quiet and still. Become aware of your body and how you feel right now. Feel the energy going through you and see where it takes your attention. As I mention each body part, be aware of what you are sensing in that part without thinking of it as good or bad.

Guided Visualization

The Interrelatedness of Life

Imagine a perfect world of which we are all a part and imagine yourself as an element of nature. You might be

a blade of grass

a beetle

the trunk of a tree, strong and sturdy

a running brook going over rocks

an elephant stomping through the jungle

a dolphin playfully swimming through the ocean

a kitten chasing another kitten

a flower unfolding

the branches of a tree reaching upward
    toward the sun

wind moving
    through space
        making a breeze
            on a hot summer day

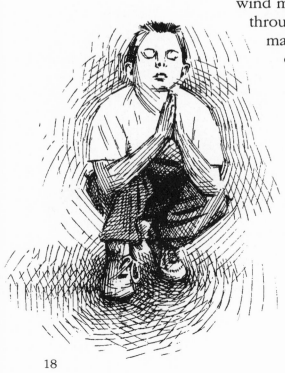

rain washing the earth, the rocks and the air

a huge leaf protecting some small creature in the rain forest

birds soaring through the sky freely, wings spread wide, gliding to a rock in the ocean or the branch of a tree

You may have another image that is a part of life and growth and change.

Movement

Using the image you chose, let it take over your body little by little. Feel it in your
    face
        head
           neck
               shoulders
                  arms
                     legs
                       torso

Feel your nature image fully.
    Now let your body feel and move as if it were this part of nature.
I invite you to move throughout the room using its qualities.
    soft
        swift
           strong
              gentle
not touching any other person.
    Be aware of the boundaries of other living things.
Acknowledge the other as you dance toward each life form you encounter.
    Present yourself in your dance as if in a conversation with other parts of nature.
Be fully who you are as you acknowledge your new partner.
    Move freely from life form to life form, admiring the beauty and uniqueness of
each part of nature.
    Each new life form you come to will stimulate and inspire new shapes and
movements in you.
    Dance with as many other parts of nature as you can.
In slow motion come together as closely as possible. Without
touching, freeze the position so that we can tell if you are
    a huge rock
      a bird
        a cat
          rain
another part of nature.

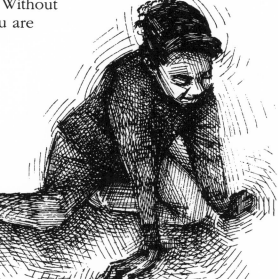

    In this frozen moment of time, take a look
around and observe the beauty of us all
together, coexisting in one world.
    You will be standing in this position
for about five minutes. Adjust your
position so that you can stay
comfortable.
    If anyone gets tired and
needs a chair, let me know.

***Once a child asked for a chair, stood on it, and
said that he was the sun, watching over everyone.***

Creating the Web

Now we need webmakers. Those of you who chose not to be part of nature can now help us make the web. You will be given rolls of streamers of different colors. People of the web, you can choose to come out of the web and be the webmakers instead.

This is a good opportunity to include children who did not want to participate. I have offered them a colorful roll of crepe paper and asked if they would help us make the web. Because they become interested through observation and have been enjoying the process, this gesture often gets everyone fully involved.

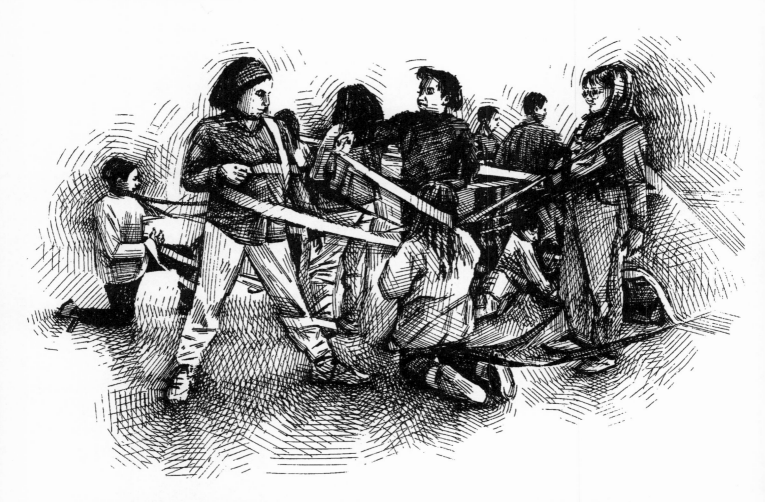

Webmakers, hand the end of your roll of crepe paper to one child to hold and then, moving in and out through the other children, wind the crepe paper around, under and over their arms, legs, shoulders and so forth. Be careful not to wind it around the neck. Everyone likes to watch the web being created, so don't cover anyone's eyes. Webmakers, as other children are winding their colors through the group, you may have to step over or under the other streamers. When you have finished your roll of paper, give the end to someone to hold or tuck it into another's pocket or sleeve.

Now that the webmakers have finished making the web, you can move in and out and over and under the spaces of the web you have created.

Webmakers can now take a special place in the web. You may sit on the floor and look up at it from below;

you may stand in one of the spaces;

you may take the shape of a part of nature and be part of the web.

Now we can move in slow motion, each of us affecting the web and one another with our movement.

Remember to move very slowly so we don't break the web.

Naming

The web includes all living things.

One at a time, I would like you to tell the others who you are and say a few words or a sentence about yourself. I will not tell you when it is your turn. You will have to be aware of each other and not talk at the same time. You will each know when it is your turn. If you choose, you may build upon the ideas of others.

One group of children who built upon each other's ideas said

I am a flowing river.

I am a seagull soaring over the river.

I am the wind moving wherever I want to go.

I am the storm that is creating the wind.

I am a kangaroo jumping in the wind.

I am a lion chasing the kangaroo.

You are all beautiful parts of nature

connected to each other

dependent on each other

giving to each other

related to each other

growing with each other.

While we are all connected to the web we can sing a song.
Sing "Let There Be Peace on Earth."

We come together and we are separate.

In leaving today please take a part of the web with you.

Art

We will make a large mural of all your nature ideas.

So Long and Hello

One person is moving away and leaving our class so we will say good-bye in a special way. We want her to know that we still want to be connected.

Marge may stand in the center holding different colored crepe paper streamers. Each one of us will take one color and unravel it as we connect it to ourselves in different ways as well as drape it around Marge. It almost looks like a maypole with Marge as the center.

Each of us can say something to Marge as we connect ourselves to her. We might say, for example,

"Marge, we wish you a good journey."
"We hope you make lots of friends in your new school."
"I wish you good luck in your new home."
"I hope you will remember us for we will miss you."

We can also do this to welcome a new classmate, saying such things as,
"We are glad you are here and we want you to be our friend."

UNDERSTANDING DIFFERENCES

Discussion

How are we different?
    We have different
        faces
            names
                talents
                    personalities
How else are we different from each other?

Supporting differences as a positive part of ourselves is very important, as some children experience their differences from others as negative; racial minorities, for instance, often feel negative about their differences in our society.

Art

We will draw pictures of ourselves. These will be feeling pictures, so you don't have to worry about how they are going to look, or whether they are exact likenesses. We will put these pictures around the room and everyone may stand next to his or her picture. Those who choose to can say something about themselves and how they feel different from everyone else.

Photographic History

Bring in photographs of yourself at different ages. We will place them in chronological order and you can see how you changed as you grew older.

Hiding

Do you think you have something different that no one knows about? Something you feel you need to hide or keep private?

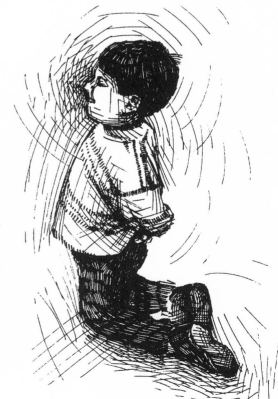

You don't have to tell us about your differences, but let's explore how it feels to have a secret.

Sit across from a partner. I would like one of you to hide your elbow from your partner. Partner, gently try to see the hidden elbow. Don't leave your seat. Be aware of how you are feeling while you hide your elbow.

Get ready to show your elbow, and be aware of how you are feeling right now. Show your elbow to your partner. Partner, be supportive and caring. This may be a difficult moment for the person who is hiding an elbow.

How do you feel now, after you have shown your elbow?

Reverse roles.

Take a few minutes to talk to your partner about how you felt hiding and showing your elbow in the three stages of hiding, getting ready to show and showing.

Some Responses

Hiding

Felt trapped, strained, knot in stomach, embarrassed, nervous, scared, wondered how it would be to show your secret.

Getting Ready

Felt scared, silly, afraid, didn't know how other person would react, happy, embarrassed, daring, confused.

Showing

Felt relieved, no longer frustrated.

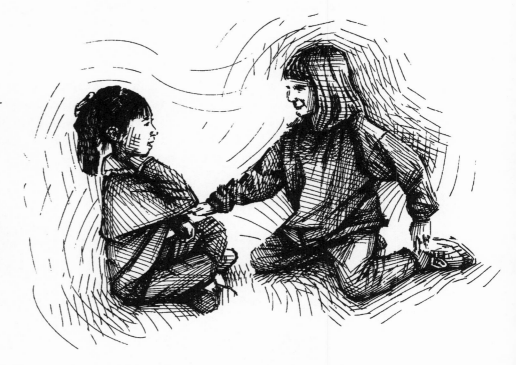

The usual response is that it is easier to be with people when they are not always hiding something about themselves. The discussion evolved to other people they knew who had outstanding differences, and then some of the children shared their secrets. Children should not feel pressured to reveal their secrets. Following is an example of one group of children that shared.

> *I have dyslexia.*
>> Can you explain what that is?
>>> *I have problems reading. I sometimes read words backward.*

A third grader helped us pronounce this difficult word.

A first-grade child said, *When I was born, my lung was collapsed and the doctor had to operate on me. I still have a scar on my chest. You can see it when I go swimming. People stare at me.*

"How do you feel to be stared at?"

I don't like it.

A mainstreamed fourth-grade child with cerebral palsy said, *I have a disability.*

"What is your disability?"

With tremendous effort and power, this little girl, who was much smaller than most of the other children, said, *Well, I wear two kinds of braces. One is for my leg and another is for my foot and I have problems with my left hand.*

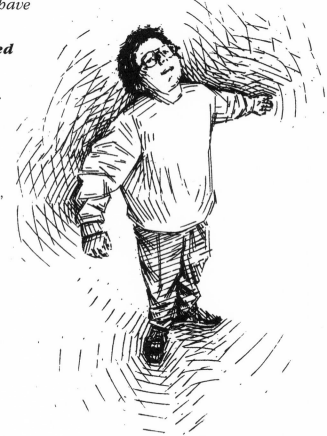

All of the children spontaneously applauded this little girl.

Another child said, *I have a wetting problem. I wet the bed too much.*

"Does anyone else have that problem?"

Six others raised their hands. "That's the kind of problem you can usually outgrow. Thank you for sharing all of that with us today."

Warm Fuzzies

We will now give one child at a time a chance to get good strokes.

Angie can come up and we will say all of the wonderful things we can think of about Angie.

Everything positive and nice, using one word or short sentences.

Permanent Feedback

We can make a huge poster of these words and phrases so that you can take it home to remind yourselves of how wonderful you are.

We can also tape it so you can listen to it whenever you need positive feedback.

After everyone has had a turn you can ask, "How does it feel to have something nice said about you?" Give me one-word answers.

marvelous	*awesome*	*decent*	*perfect*
splendid	*happy*	*proud*	*super*
dynamite	*exploding*	*fine*	*glad*
gleeful	*wonderful*	*good*	*terrific*
flattered	*outstanding*	*fantastic*	*great*
tremendous	*the kid of the class*		

Now you will move around the room as I say these words, allowing your body to express the way these words make you feel.

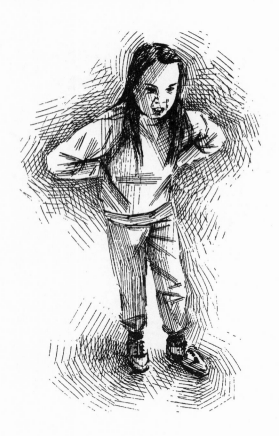

How would you feel if you were teased?

Call out some one word answers.

ashamed	*crying*
upset	*left out*
angry	*lonely*
lousy	*bad*
horrible	*disturbed*
sad	*traumatized*
hurt	*crumbling*
insulted	

Move around the room while I say these words, and let your body react to them.

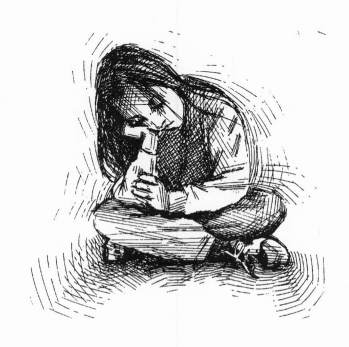

Masks

Create a mask that shows how you are feeling. You can use oak tag or papier mâché.

Some feelings may be
Scary
Beautiful
Brave
Terrible
Happy
Sad
Terrific

Using the mask, you may dance the feeling it represents.
Exchange masks with someone and dance the new feeling.
Exchange again and dance that feeling.

Younger children can paste different shapes and materials on oak tag that was previously cut in the shape of a mask.

Imagery

Make yourself comfortable and close your eyes. Visualize a lovely place you would like to be. It may be a forest, the beach, the mountains, your home or any other place of your choosing. Any time of year. The warmth of the summer, the newness of spring, the briskness and colors of autumn, the cold and whiteness of winter. How are you dressed? What are you doing? How are you doing it? What is the surface of the ground like? How does it feel to you? Enjoy yourself thoroughly.

After a while you will see someone in the distance slowly coming toward you. As this person comes closer still, you notice that he or she is about the same size, age and sex as you are. You realize that this person is extremely attractive but you haven't recognized this person yet. As this person moves even closer you realize that he or she is you. Enjoy being with her or him realizing how much you like yourself. I will count to three for you to open your eyes. One. Begin to feel the ground underneath you and be aware of where you are. Two. Begin to stretch your arms and legs. Three. Open your eyes slowly and be aware of your feelings.

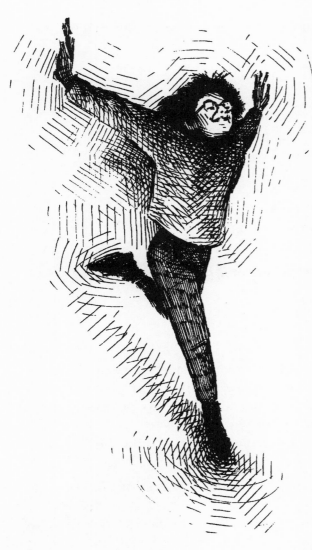

Dance Me Beautiful

Use inspiring music such as Ravel's Bolero.

Dance to the music as I tell you your story. Feel the beautiful you! Feel your beauty in your toes, in your legs, throughout your body, up your neck, into your head and down your arms. Your whole beautiful self is dancing. Make a statement with your dance. Saying, "I am beautiful. I am great. I am wonderful." Move throughout the room, making your statement and being your unique self. Be as only you can be.

Dancing You.

Look at all of the different and unique beauties. As you move throughout the room, stop when you reach someone and dance with that person. Introduce yourself without talking, and show off your beauty to the other person. Keep your unique style as you share yourself. Move on to another person.

Dance your beauty with that person and then move on, meeting as many beautiful people as you can.

Writing

Go back to your portrait. On it write some words that describe you. Take another piece of paper and make up some sentences using those words, creating a story about yourself.

It can be real or imaginary. Those who would like to can share their stories in small groups or with the whole class.

Some children may enjoy making up stories about each other.

Some of these stories can be dramatized. Children can act out parts spontaneously as the story is being told.

For younger children these stories can be shared verbally rather than written down.

Showing Off

Let's make a large circle. One at a time you will go into the center and create a beautiful sculpture that represents you. We will all appreciate you. You may use scarves or the large pieces of silk fabric to aid you in your dance.

Yes, that's great! Now the next person, and the next, until all who would like have danced.

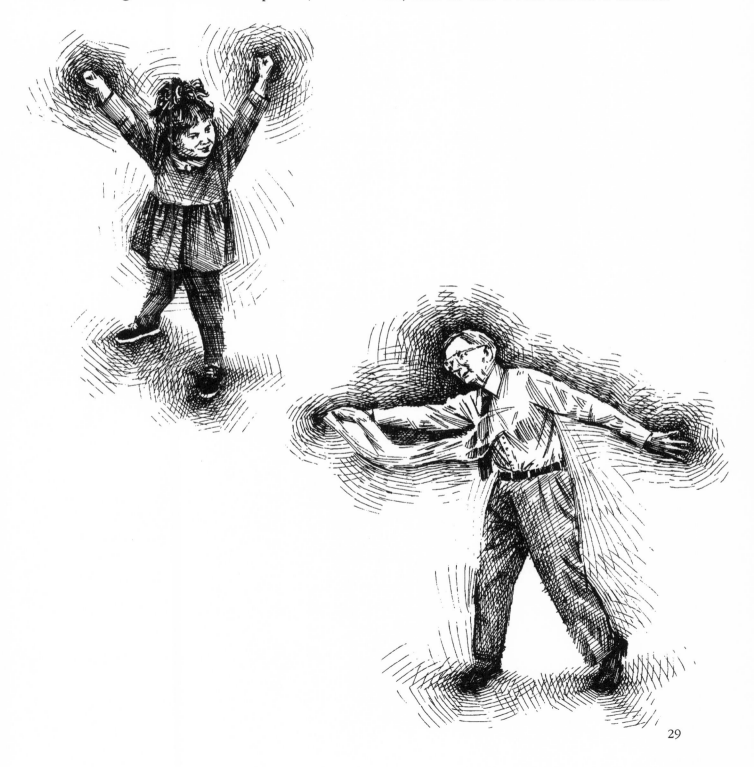

Weave the Ring

Still in a circle, every other person face right and the others face left. We will move, taking each other's hands, first the left and then the right, around and around while I say these words:

We are all beautiful.
    We are all unique.
        We are all different.
            And we are all together.
                We need to touch each other,
                    teach each other,
                        learn from each other,
                            and care for each other.

We are all in one world,
    different and same,
        separate and together.

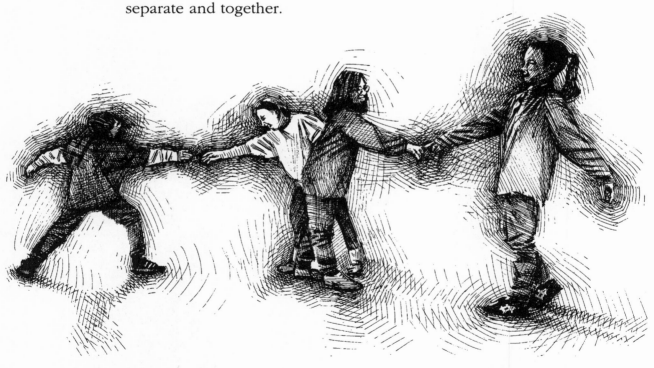

You may say things about yourself as you weave around such as:
I have brown hair, I have blue eyes, I love to dance, I am good at basketball.

Snake Around

Come into the circle again. I will drop my hand and snake around the circle as the rest of you follow. I will be facing each person as I pass.

Make eye contact as you pass each of your friends.

We will celebrate our uniqueness and respect the uniqueness in others.

I am bringing our snake dance into a tight spiral, tightening inward, around and around, until there is no more room to move.

We are in a tight circle bunched together.

We are different and we are one.

Now relax and spread out a little so you can sit down.

Tell us how you are feeling.

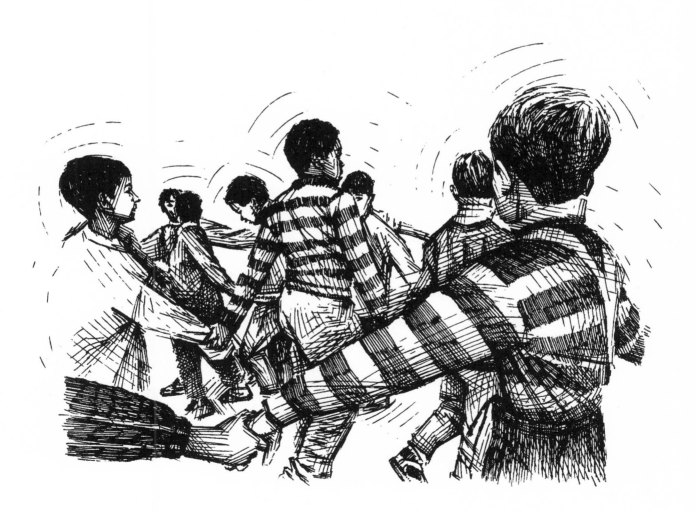

Animals

Pick an animal that represents the part of yourself that your mask hides. Feel that animal in all parts of your body and begin to move, staying in our circle. One at a time you may come into the center and be that animal. If you give your permission, we will guess who you are. If you choose, you may tell the others why you picked that animal.

Would you like to share your animal?

Some examples were:

I am a monkey. People think I kid around too much.
I am a gazelle. People think I'm stuck-up.
I am a boa constrictor because I squeeze people too much.

Let's have the animals interact with one another. Let's play and enjoy each other as animals.

Now that we have experienced the animal we usually like to hide, can you find something positive to say about your animal? Say it in the first person.

I am a monkey that enjoys having fun.
I am a graceful gazelle.
I am a boa constrictor that can wind around in a very smooth and powerful way and am a really good hugger.

Great! Everyone who wants to may share.

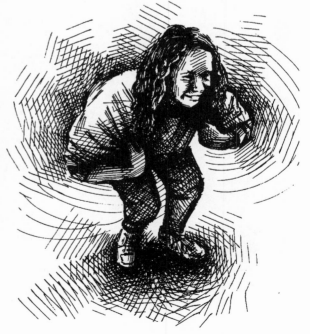

Variations

Choose animals to reflect your inner self and how you see yourself. Choose an animal that reflects how you think others see you.

Fantasy Art

Draw yourselves as the animal you most admire. That may look like some combination of parts of yourself and parts of the animal. Draw it any way you like. It's your fantasy.

Project Feeling Sculptures

Sculpt your partner into what you think your partner is thinking about you. Share your thoughts with your partner and then get his feedback.

Were you right about what you thought?

How different were your partner's feelings about you?

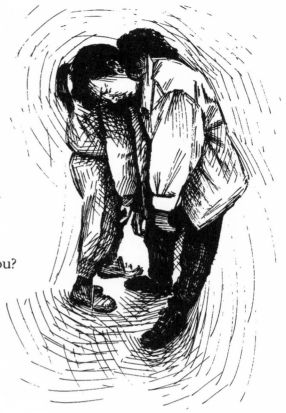

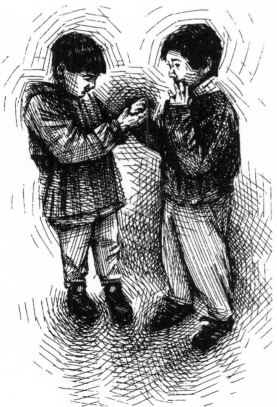

Nonverbal Communication

Differences: Hand Conversation

Walk around the room looking for someone you think is your opposite. Choose that person as your partner.

Communicate with your partner using your hands only.

Show strength, playfulness, fright, fighting, friendship, caution.

Now let your hands dance.

Take some time to tell each other why you think you may be opposites and whether you still think you are.

Can you communicate with another part of your body?

How about expressing sadness or caring with your head?

Same: Mirroring

Now walk around the room looking for someone you think is the same as you. Choose that person as your partner.

One of you will be the leader, and the other will mirror exactly what the leader is doing. Leader, move slowly so that your partner can follow you. Each of you will experience what it is to move as the other. Mirror, is the movement familiar? Is this the way you normally move? Now change roles.

Share with your partner why you first felt you were the same and whether you still feel that way.

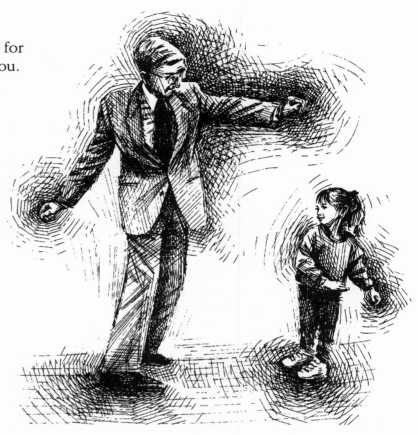

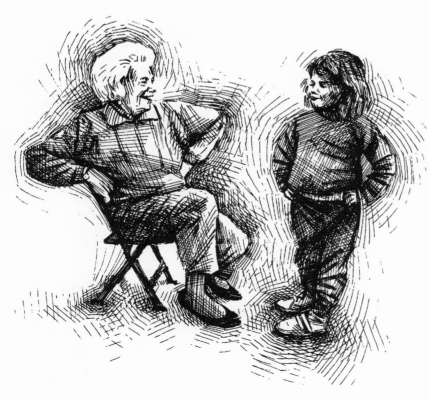

Movement activities such as mirroring can be enjoyed by all ages. Some organizations have understood the importance of bringing the elderly and young children together to offer an invaluable experience for both. The seniors appreciate and enjoy new life and energy from the children as well as feel needed as the children enjoy the wisdom, support and nurturing from the elderly.

Conflict: Yes-No dance

Walk around the room looking for someone you think might be in conflict. Choose that person as a partner.

One of you will be yes and one will be no. Use only your body to take turns expressing yes and no. Make it a conversation, one answering the other. This can be fun. How many ways can you show yes and no?

Now change roles so that you can experience the opposite.

Share your reactions to this experience with your partner.

Reactions to yes were:
> *It felt easy*
> > *I got to jump up and down.*

Reactions to no were:
> *Easier to be no because someone had to beg, you*
> > *get to refuse, I learned to say no, don't have*
> > > *to get refused, was able to say no to*
> > > > *someone older than you.*

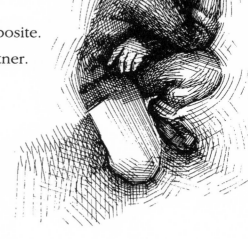

Cooperation with Yes and No

Begin at opposites sides of the room. Mover yes and mover no create a dance saying yes or no in different ways.

Now begin to move toward the middle of the room toward each other.

As you get closer, begin to change your movements so that no begins to look like yes and yes begins to look like no and start mirroring each other. Allow your movements to flow back and forth from yes movements to no movements. Yes and no are beginning to cooperate in this way.

We have all experienced similar emotions.

I would like everyone to walk through the space reacting to the following words:

powerful	weak
playful	sad
courageous	frightened
lovable	shy

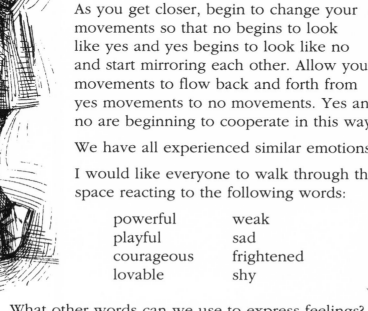

What other words can we use to express feelings?

Follow the Leader

One person will lead the rest of the group in expressing a feeling. We will all try to express that feeling in our own way.

When I call someone's name, that person will become the leader and show us a new feeling that we will all express, each in our own way.

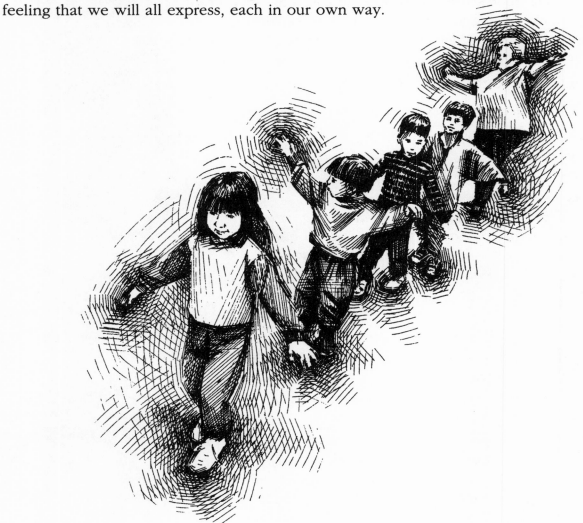

Homework Assignment

Find three people each day, seven days a week, and say something nice to them. One of these people can be you, but please face yourself in the mirror when you say something nice to yourself. One of these people might be someone in your class or your family. It might be someone who helped you in a store, or someone who is very old or very young. Maybe someone with a disability or who looks very different from you.

An immediate reaction to this homework assignment has been that many of the children put an arm around the shoulders of the child next to them and give a little squeeze. Everyone smiles. They seem to feel very good about one another.

T R A N S I T I O N S

Becoming
  growing
    evolving
      maturing
        progressing
          developing
            unfolding
              transforming
                changing
                  improving

Life is a continuous metamorphosis of becoming,
knowing and living all our internal characters
so that we can enjoy and delight in
an exciting and rewarding experience.

MOTHER'S DAY
AND FATHER'S DAY

Music: (Lullaby from the Womb)

Guided Imagery

Get into a comfortable sleeping position. It's been a long, cold winter and you want to stay warm and cuddled up, safe in your own world.

Listen to the rhythm of your heartbeat.

Is it your heartbeat?
Is it the heartbeat of your parent?
Is it the heartbeat of the Earth?
The rhythm of all nature?
Is it the same?
Is it part of all of us?
Are we all part of nature?

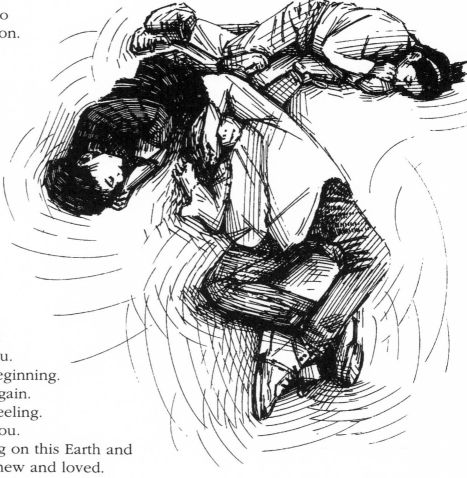

Let your body roll over into another comfortable position. While you're cuddled and sleeping, you are having ideas, thoughts and fantasies. These ideas, feelings and fantasies need more room, so let your body roll over to another comfortable position. Allow your thoughts and feelings to be free and flow through you. And while you lie so protected and warm, you can feel loved.

Full of hopes and dreams. You are perfect and I can't wait to see and be with you.

You are in a new beginning.
You're starting again.
It is a good feeling.
It is just you.
You are an important being on this Earth and
you feel secure, fresh, new and loved.

Rolling and Stretching

Just feel the comfort and very slowly reach out . . .
   uncurling softly in no special way . . .
      begin to stretch your arms in all directions.

Feel the freedom of your movements . . .
   Let your fingers explore the air . . .
      "Oh! how wonderfully my arms and hands can move," you say to yourself . . .
    What is this new feeling?

Bring your shoulders into the movement. Let your arms encircle your head and reach and stretch and twist and circle and twine around, exploring all the space around you from your seated position.

Begin to watch the patterns in the air your arms and hands are making.

Look at your arms as if for the first time and think: "Look at these beautiful arms I have that are making these marvelous patterns!"

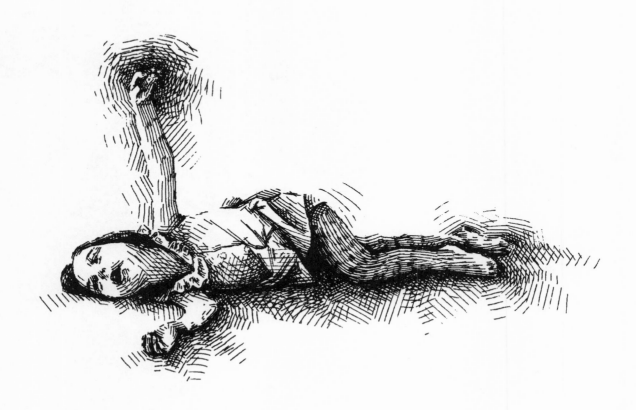

Group Awareness

Now let's use more room.
　　Let your body roll.
　　　　Begin to let your eyes meet the eyes of others.
　　　　　　Ah! I am not alone.
　　　　　　　　I am not the only one.
　　　　　　　　　　There are others with me.

Move toward these other friends.

There is lots of space to explore and lots of friends are rolling with you. Gently, slowly, roll with new friends, greeting them only with your body as you may bump into each other and have to change direction. Be gentle when you come upon another friend who is also rolling.

Let your body roll over to yet another comfortable position and begin a slow stretch . . . a slow waking up of your body, a slow waking up of your mind, a nice stretch of your imagination.

There are others here. You are not alone. Share your larger space. Continue stretching, letting your whole body stretch itself into a sitting position.

Allow one body part after another to stretch and twist and awaken. Only your body will tell you which part wants to twist and stretch. Listen to it. You may want to stretch with a friend who is close to you. Use each other to help the parts of your body stretch.

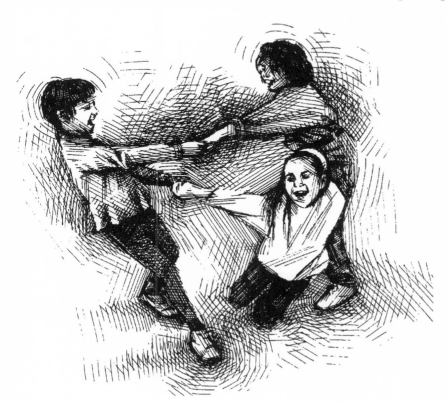

Slowly rise, twisting, turning and rolling up, until you are standing.

For Children with Special Needs
by Louise Kelsey

We are going to roll you into a flannel sheet and gently pressure you from the outside, helping you roll.

This activity will give a tactile defensive child sensory stimulation. It is nonthreatening because it is not direct touch.

Awakening

Keeping eyes lowered, turn toward the nearest person for a partner and sit down facing each other.

Quietly look into each other's face. It is a brand new world.

Look into the loving, kind eyes of another human being.

Be there quietly with each other.

Feel nice thoughts flowing between you.

Acknowledge the kindness and caring you are giving and getting in some way.

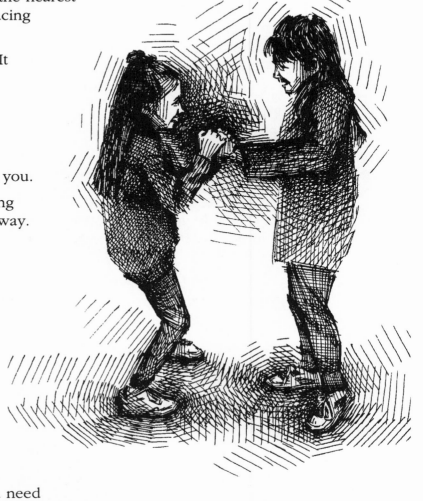

Sharing Gifts
(Music: "From Thee I Receive")

This is make-believe. You will be giving your partner gifts of life from Mother Nature. Take turns giving gifts without talking. Receive the gift and place it somewhere. Then take your turn giving. The gifts may be real, such as a sip of water or imaginary, such as a shower of stars. All are fantasy. You need not know what you are giving or receiving to appreciate the feeling of giving and receiving.

Michael, age four, who had difficulty pretending, did a cartwheel, dance or somersault for his gift.

For Children with Special Needs

Brenda, who has Down's syndrome, is a very responsive child. While the partners were giving gifts, she spontaneously turned to other children to give them gifts. This stimulated other children to change partners independently, moving from one to the next and giving one another gifts. This was an opportunity to expand an activity by using the children's spontaneity, turning it into another creative and involved activity, with little structure imposed by adults.

Rocking
(Music: Pachelbel's Canon in D)

Become a group of four.

Three of you may find a way to take your fourth partner gently into your arms. Take turns being nurtured, cuddled and rocked as if you were a newborn baby. Feel your newness. Look at your fingers and toes as a newborn child.

Each group take the newborn into your loving arms.

Say I love you.
  I will clothe you.
    I will blanket you.
      I will protect you.
        I will look into your sweet face.
       I will feed you.
        I will nurture you.

I will see you.
  I will be with you.
    I will care for you.
      We welcome you to the world.
      Welcome you to the universe.
      To the great outdoors.
       To be with loving people.
        We welcome you to life.
         We welcome your beauty.

your joy
  your love
    your intelligence.

You are a sweet, beautiful child.

Say whatever else you can think of that will make your baby feel good, cared for and happy to be here.

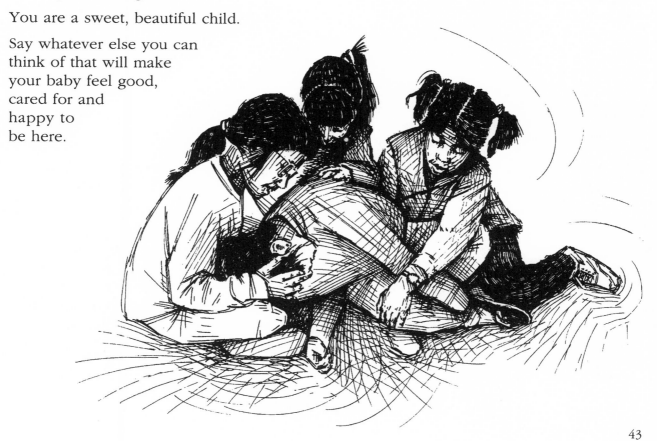

For Children with Special Needs

We will welcome the child into the world by putting him or her into a flannel blanket. The rest of your group can gently swing your child.

This activity gives the child tactile feedback and a way of experiencing an infant's feelings.

Bolster
by Louise Kelsey

Some children can straddle a bolster to experience the rocking while their growing tolerance for physical proximity is respected.

Descriptive Words

Think of one word to describe your mother, father and child. A fourth grade class gave these responses:

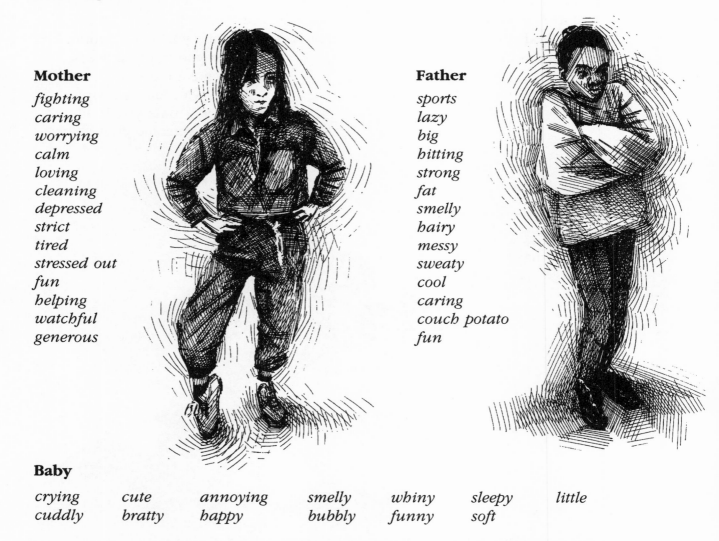

Mother

fighting
caring
worrying
calm
loving
cleaning
depressed
strict
tired
stressed out
fun
helping
watchful
generous

Father

sports
lazy
big
hitting
strong
fat
smelly
hairy
messy
sweaty
cool
caring
couch potato
fun

Baby

crying	*cute*	*annoying*	*smelly*	*whiny*	*sleepy*	*little*
cuddly	*bratty*	*happy*	*bubbly*	*funny*	*soft*	

This exercise provides a lot of information about how children see their own parents and parental roles. You can take it further with storytelling, writing and discussion about how some qualities fit both mothers and fathers.

Movement

How does your mother or father walk?
  Show us.

Be your mother or father in the living room,
  at the barbecue,
    at a family gathering or party.

Where else would you like to be your parent?

Think of some things you see your mother or father doing.

Act them out and let us guess.

I'm glad to see boys taking Mom roles and girls taking Dad roles, as well as the other way around.

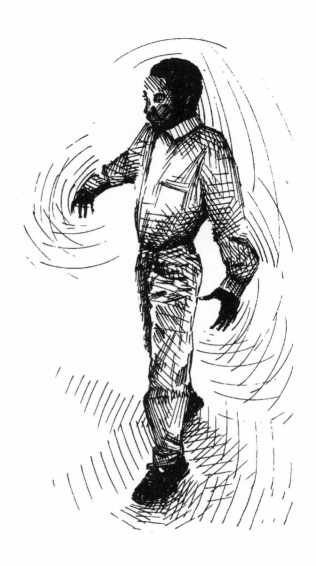

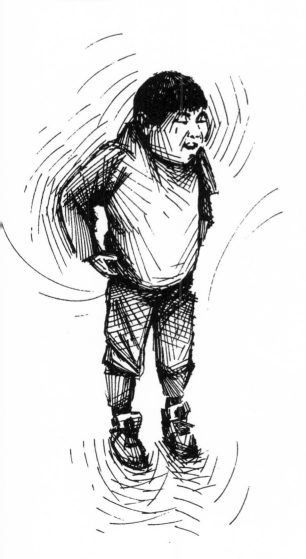

The Dance

Decide whether you want to be the father, mother or baby dancing through the room in that role. Let your movements fully become a dance and now freeze. Wow! Look at all the different types of mommies, daddies and babies.

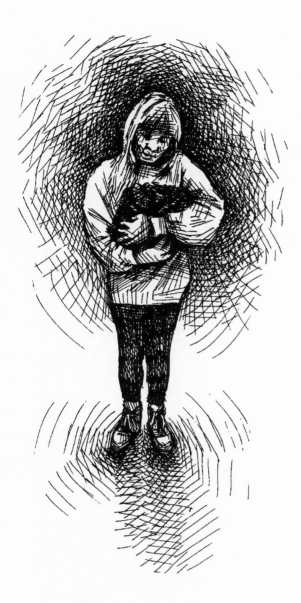

You Are the Parent

Be your mother or father, holding a doll or rolled-up towel or blanket that is you.

*Have some lullabies
or soothing music playing.*

Rock your baby softly.
Hum to your baby.
Tell your baby that she or he is
beautiful or handsome.
Say the following things after me.
You are smart.
You are lovable.
You are sweet.
You are good.
You are wonderful.
You are precious.
What else would you like to say to your child?

Positive Feedback

Think of the most wonderful thing your mother or father could say to you. Something marvelous that you would like very much to hear.

Half of you sit in a comfortable, cuddled position with your eyes closed. The other half will act as the mother or father and move around the room, whispering that positive, wonderful thing to each child.

Now switch roles so that everyone can experience this positive event.

Let's all sit in a circle. Those who would like to can orally share their feelings with the others.

Fantasy Playmate

Imagine a picture book. The cover is very colorful. You open it. You see a wide, open field with green grass and flowers. The sky is spacious with big fluffy clouds, a feeling of newness. Turn the page. The same scene. In the middle of the grass is a child your age, asleep. Gently awaken the child.

What would you like to do with your playmate? Provide him or her with anything he or she may want. Maybe you want to run or skip or play ball. Have fun and enjoy yourselves. I will be silent for a few moments while you weave your story.

Sculpture

Pick two other children to be your parents.

You may choose to have one parent,
a grandparent, a foster parent or any
person you feel close to in your family.

Position them in a group as you normally see them.
Sculpt them in ways you would like to see them.
Place yourself in the sculpture with your family.
Try different positions.
Add other family members in your sculpture.

***For more instructions see Passive/Active
in* A Moving Experience, *page 110.***

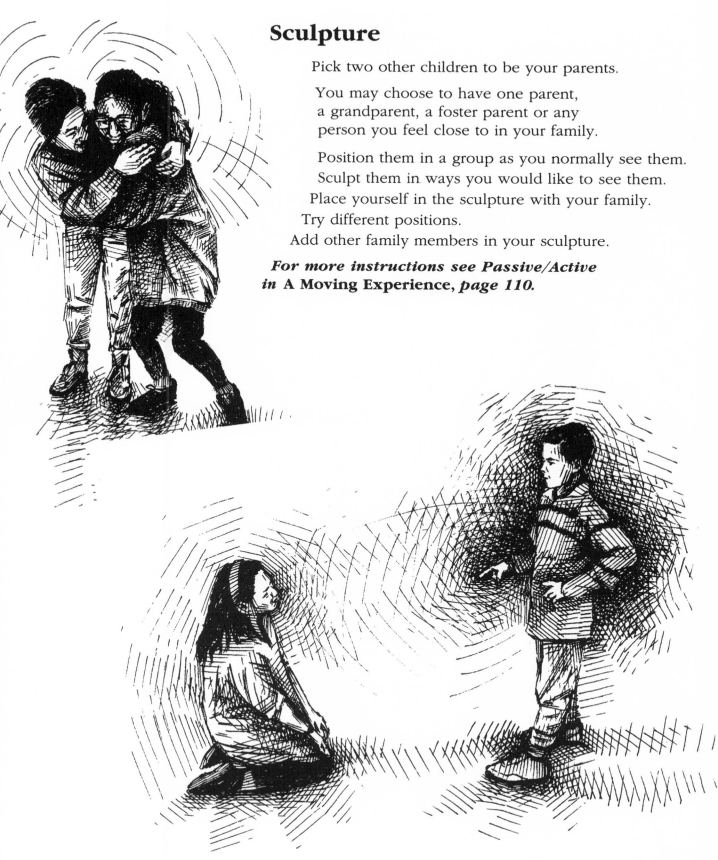

Sharing

What would you like to say about your family sculpture?
> Describe who is in your picture and tell us what they are doing.
> > Some may be objects such as tables, chairs and doors.

Don't forget your pets!
> You may have them interacting with or ignoring one another.

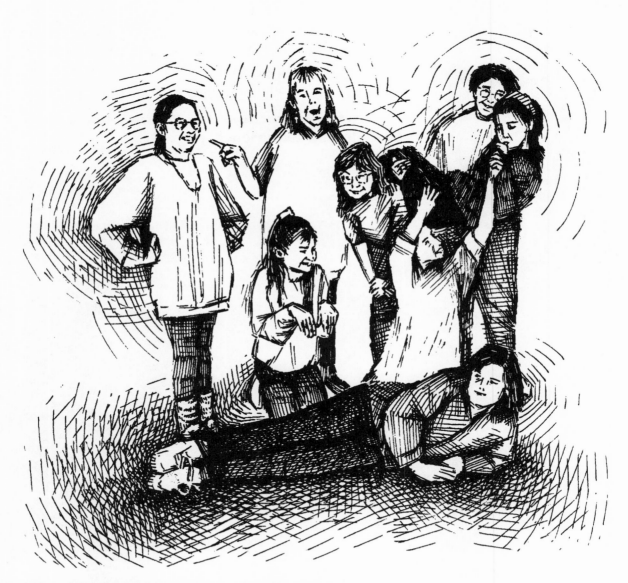

Descriptions shared in this particular group:

Dog begging
Teenager watching television
Father reading
Uncle watching

Mom yelling at daughter who
   is supposed to be cleaning
Sister waving
A table

Relaxation

We will now pair up as parent and child.

Child, begin by lying down on your back, stretched out, as relaxed as possible. Parent, very gently take your child's head in your hands and as slowly as possible, move it from side to side.

Try moving his head even slower.

Child, don't help your parent by lifting your head. Allow your parent to hold the full weight of your head.

Now change positions. The parent may trust the child to hold her head and do the same.

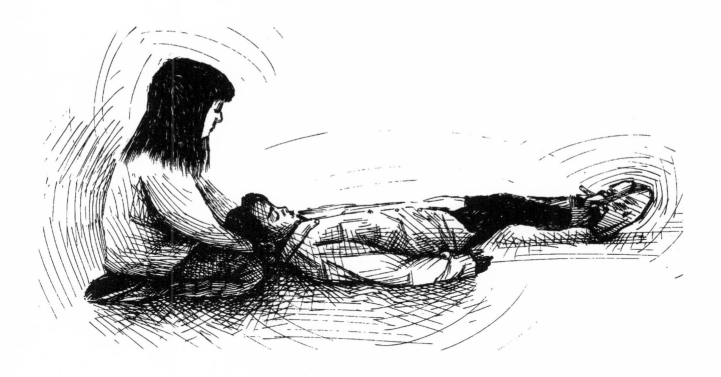

Sharing

Partners may talk about the shared experience for a few minutes. Tell your partner whether you were able to feel trust. Tell whether you felt he or she was trusting you. How did it feel to trust and be trusted? Did you feel tense or relaxed?

Mother's and Father's Day Cards

My mom's/dad's name is _____

Her/His favorite color is _____

She/He loves to eat _____

She/He looks the prettiest/handsomest when _____

She/He spends most of her/his time _____

My mom/dad is very smart. She/He knows all about _____

Whenever we're together, this is what I like to do best _____

My mom/dad is the best mom/dad in the world because _____

One of the things I like about my mom/dad is _____

My mom/dad is always in charge of _____

I feel special when my mom/dad does _____

Add your own thoughts to the list.

Art

Draw a picture or write some of your feelings or thoughts now.

Collage

Look through some magazines to find pictures of things your mother or father would enjoy or things that remind you of your mother or father.

Cut them out and make a collage.

Cut the outside of your collage into an interesting shape without destroying the pictures. Paste the collage on a large sheet of construction paper and give it as a present for Mother's or Father's Day.

You may want to combine your drawing and collage to create one picture.

THE EGG
AND THE CHICKEN

Visualization

Everyone, find your own space on the floor, not too close to each other and not too close to walls or furniture.

Close your eyes so that you can see the picture I'm about to describe.

We are going to make believe that you are an unborn chicken, still inside the protective egg. Curl yourself up to be as small as possible.

I will ask you some questions. Answer them in your head without talking. Some of the things I will ask you, you will be able to try, and some you will think about or fantasize.

Questions

Is it warm or cold inside the egg?
Is it wet or dry?
Is it sticky?
      How does that feel?
Is the inside of your eggshell rough or smooth?
Is it light or dark?
Is it hard or soft?
      What do you like about it?
Is there anything else inside with you?
What colors do you see?
Tap on the shell very lightly so that it
won't crack.
      What does it sound like?
What does it smell like?
Does it smell sweet or sour?
Can you wiggle inside? Try it.
Can you stretch,
  twist,
    turn,
      rock,
        shake,
          roll,
            or sit up?

See if you can do those movements
or any other without breaking the shell.

Coming Out

You are now old enough to leave your eggshell.

Very gently, with your beaks, begin to crack open your shell.
Do so slowly and little by little, until you can come out into the open.

   How are you feeling as you come out for the first time?
Are you excited about the new world?
   Are you feeling shy? Do you want to go back into the shell?
Remember, you are newborn and very little.
   How will you move around as a newborn chick?
Move your head slowly and look at the new world.
   What do you see that interests you?
Try your wings. Move them slowly, now faster and faster.

Now slow down to a stop. Try your little thin legs. They might be wobbly at first, so you'll have to move around the room very slowly. You might fall over, but you will be able to get up again. Come wobble over to mother hen (teacher).

Make sure every child feels he or she has successfully come out of the shell. If they seem to be having discomfort you can help them by giving them oral support such as saying, "Come on, you can do it. Push harder. You're strong! keep pushing!" You may ask if they have a suggestion as to how you can help get them out. We can't physically help chickens out for if we do they will die. Chickens have to be strong enough to get out themselves.

Although this is imaginary play it needs to be taken seriously as it evokes real feelings.

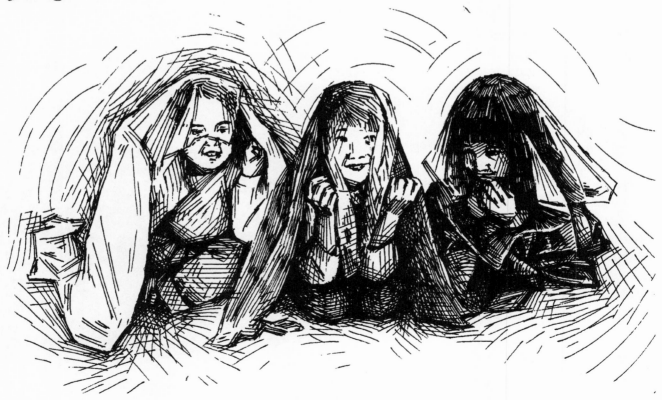

Discussion

How did it feel to be inside an egg?

Responses from Second Graders
> *Warm*
> *Shy*
> *Soft*
> *Scared of going into a different world*
> *Could hear the wind outside*

You may want to repeat the questions so that the children can answer them orally.

Props

Wrapping a sheet or tubular fabric around each child may enhance the feeling of being inside the egg. Some children may resist the sensation of being covered up. In this case, small scarves placed on some parts of their bodies can suggest enclosure.

Yellow scarves (feathers) can be worn inside the "egg" as preparation for emerging from it.

Art

Children can make an egg out of papier mâché using a balloon as a mold. Ask the children to use their imaginations as they paint their eggs.

Give children large egg-shaped construction paper to color, paint or use as the base for a collage.

Cut out a chicken mask. Let the children paste colored feathers on it. (You can buy dyed chicken feathers inexpensively at craft stores.)

Keep sheets or tubular fabric available for children to use in reenacting the chicken-and-egg dramatization during their free-play time. They will continually come up with new stories for it.

Variations

You may want to create a bug in the grass. **Have children cut tall blades of grass out of construction paper to paste on large oaktag.** Imagine how it feels and how you would move while pretending to be a little bug in tall grass. **You can also use a slide to provide a background of a forest or jungle that is appropriate for the particular image.**

Thanks to Christina Bothwell for the bug idea.

CATERPILLARS AND BUTTERFLIES

Crawling

Crawl on your bellies like caterpillars. How fast can you move? Look around at all the other caterpillars.

Are there different ways of crawling?

> On your tummies?
> > On your backs?
> > > On your sides?

What happens when you bump into another caterpillar?

Be careful to bump softly so you don't get hurt or hurt another.

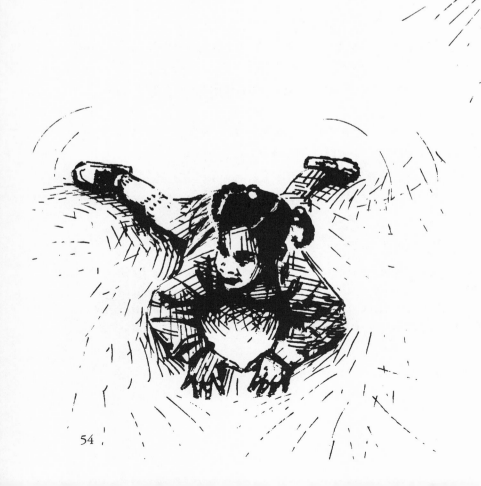

A Game

Let's play a game.

When you meet another caterpillar, each of you must turn in a different direction. Look for the empty spaces to crawl into.

Now let's change the rules for our game. When you meet another caterpillar, you have to crawl under or over each other. Do this carefully, taking good care of yourself and of each other.

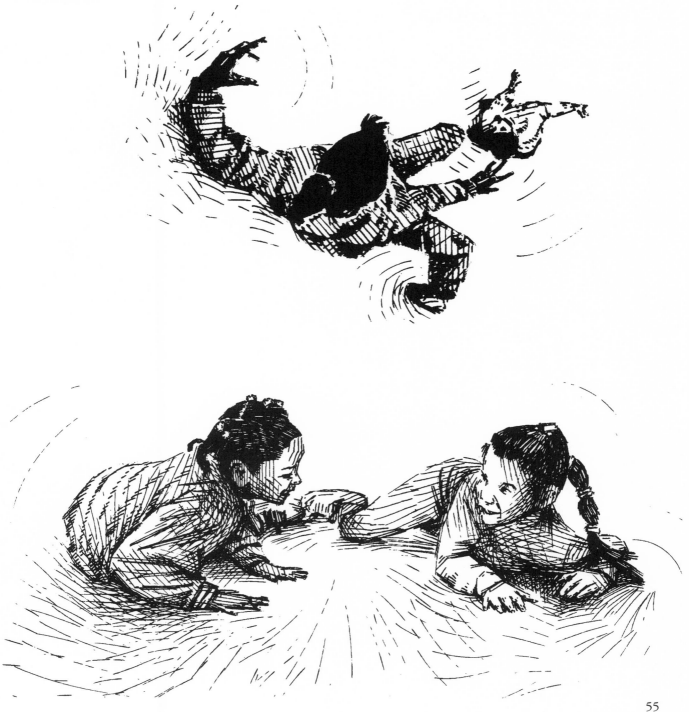

Tubular Fabric and the Butterfly

Now crawl into this long, tubular fabric. At the other end is a surprise.

As each child comes out the other end of the jersey tunnel she is handed two scarves for wings. More scarves are made available for dress-up.

Dance

Here are your beautiful wings.
  Dance with your beautiful new wings throughout the room. Now freeze.
    How do you feel?

Responses from Children

I feel beautiful.
I feel free.
I feel wonderful.
I feel as light
as air.

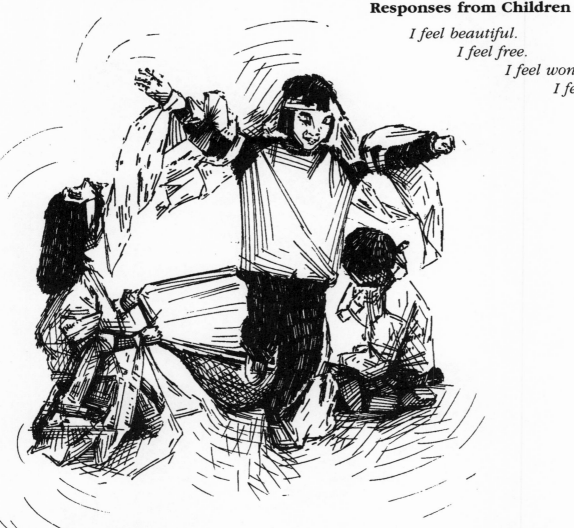

Dance freely again. Use all the space. Have fun as a beautiful free butterfly that is light as the air.

Use the children's expressed feelings by repeating them while they continue to dance.

Butterflies, you can play together. How about going under each other's wings? Using large silk fabric, two of you can make it float while other butterflies dance beneath.

Let children choose one special color for dress-up. Have them describe how that color makes them feel.

I am a beautiful red butterfly, and I feel hot. I am a lovely green butterfly, and I like the grass.

Do your dance, butterflies, and be your special color. When I say "freeze," I will ask you what you feel.

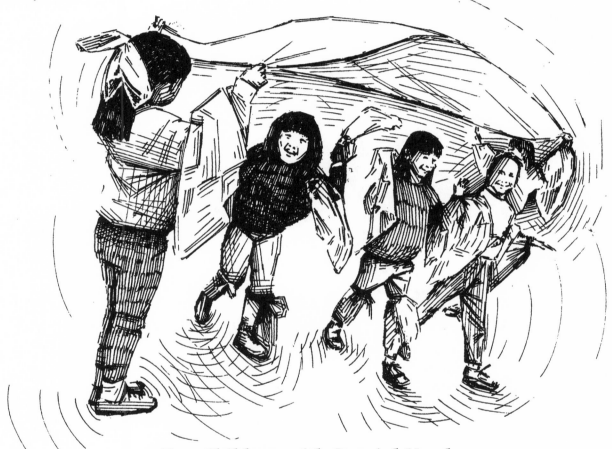

For Children with Special Needs

Let's sit around this sheet and hold the edge. The caterpillars are going under the sheet on their stomachs, backs or knees. The rest of the children will pull the sheet tight so that the caterpillars feel the sheet on top of them.

Caterpillars, when you are ready you can come out as butterflies.

The caterpillars are getting sensory stimulation all over their bodies. If a child doesn't have free motion, he can lie on a scooter and push it around under the sheet. Placing a mirror at a point of exit will give visual feedback that the child is a beautiful butterfly.

by Louise Kelsey

Art

Begin with a large butterfly shape. Paint your own beautiful butterfly.

A TREE SURVIVING
IN A CROWDED FOREST

Visualization

We will all stand together in the middle of the room. Imagine you are a tree in a very crowded forest. There are so many trees around you. Their branches are reaching for the sunlight. You also need the sun. Think of what kind of tree you are.

You may be
     gnarled,
     small,
     thick,
     leafy,
     tall
     or thin.

Allow your body to shape itself as you are imagining.

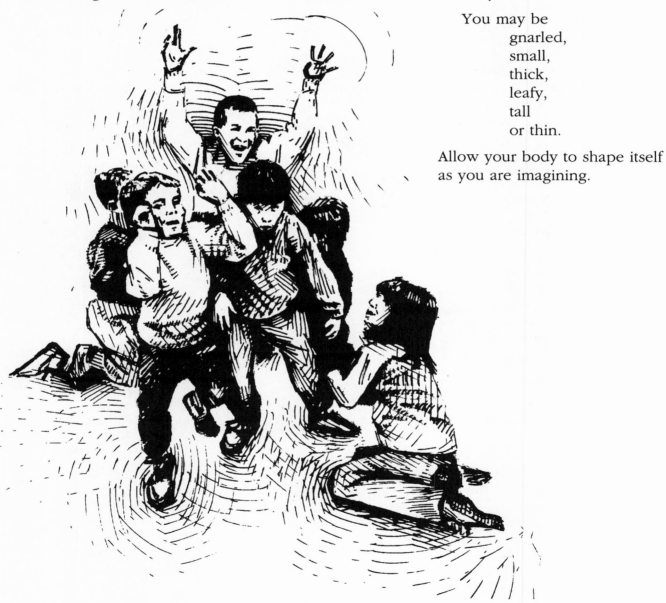

We will decide who are the strong trees that will survive and grow and who are the weak trees that will fall. You will get a chance to experience both roles. Strong trees raise your hands so we know who you are. Now the weak trees may raise their hands.

Movement

For now we will begin as a tree trunk with our arms straight by our sides. The trees are all standing close together. Very slowly your branches will try to reach up to the sun. Notice how your torso, arms and hands have to twist in different ways to find an empty space in which to rise.

Remember to do this very slowly. It takes a long time for branches to grow. Feel how difficult it is for your arms to reach out when it is so crowded.

Very slowly, the strong trees will reach for the sun. At this time you also will push very gently and firmly on the shoulders of the weak trees, making room for you to grow and receive sunlight.

Weak trees, you will slowly sink to the ground.
Strong trees, you have made it to the sun.

Because of the struggle and crowding, the branches of the strong trees will be crooked and twisted but nevertheless strong. Feel your power, strong trees. You have survived and will continue to grow.

The trees that have fallen to the ground are also an important part of nature. You will eventually go back to the earth and enrich the soil. Maybe one of your seeds will take root and grow.

Now there will be new trees growing from the seeds, and the big, strong trees will have grown old and begun to decay. At a signal, let's see the seeds slowly growing to be big strong trees and the strong trees slowly falling back down to the earth. This is done very slowly. Let's see all the different shapes of the new trees. Let's see the various shapes of trees falling to the ground and the different ways of being on the ground. Let's see how many varieties of twisted and knarled branches we can create.

Dance

Continue your movements as they become a dance. Strong trees are slowly falling back down to the earth and the new seedlings are slowly growing into strong trees.

Beautiful!

Back and forth, growing and dying and growing again. Each time try making new shapes with your body and your arms.

Charades

Be a tree in an open field, all stretched out and straight.
Be a tree in a crowded forest.

Your classmates can guess what kinds of environments you are growing in.

Be individual trees.
Be a tree that was knocked down in a windstorm.
Be a tree that has room for an animal to live in.

What animal is living with you?

Someone else may be that animal.
Could it be a squirrel, a raccoon, a woodpecker or a bluejay?
In what part of your tree is it living?
Be a tree that was chopped down for its wood.
What other kinds of trees can you think of?

Children's Responses

A tree hit by lightning
Trees eaten by termites
An apple falling off a tree
A weeping willow tree
The wind blowing the trees down
A budding tree
A redwood tree

Science

Plant a tree for Arbor Day.
Other countries and cultures also
celebrate tree planting.
In Israel they have Ta B'shevat.
In China they have Chih shee Chieh.
Japan has Greening Week.
Iceland has students of Afforestation Day.
Korea has Tree Loving Week.

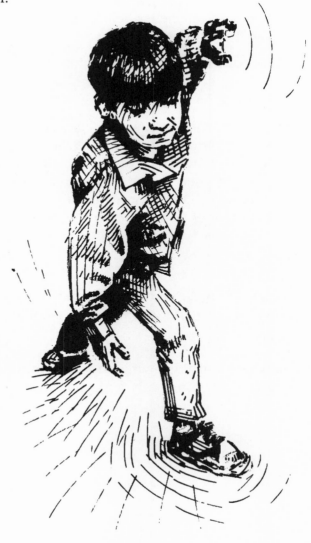

Art

Collect various twigs, leaves, flower petals, seeds and whatever else you can find on the ground to make a nature collage.

You can paste them on a sheet of oaktag or cardboard that you have already painted with your favorite colors.

In a shallow box, make an arrangement of your nature items and carefully save it.

Make a group collage. Everyone will add an object, one by one, until you have a huge collage of your nature collections.

Let's make a giant mural of a tree by painting the soles of our feet and walking up the center of the paper for the trunk.

We'll paint our hands to make hand prints for the leaves.

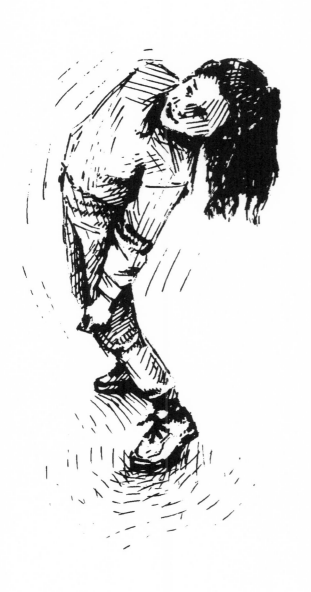
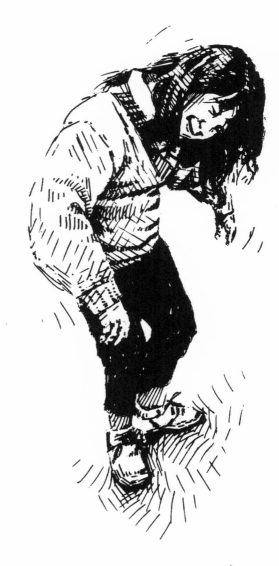

OPPOSITES

Opposites lend themselves to many
creative dance ideas and games.

Dancing the opposites gives children
a sense of themselves. Through physical
and artistic problem solving they
can develop a positive body image,
heightened self-esteem and a connection
with one another. They also become
more aware of the space around them
while learning basic concepts.

You may use these dance possibilities from
one pair of opposites to another,
by altering and adjusting as needed.

NEAR AND FAR

Body Parts

Bring your hands near your face, now send them as far as possible away from you. Lie down and bring your feet near each other. Now move them as far as possible away from each other.

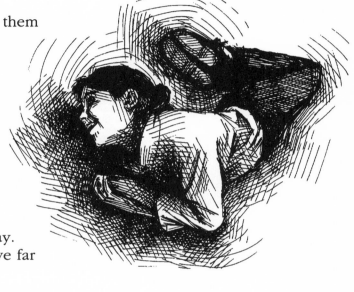

What other body parts can you move near and far from each other?

Your arms near your side and moving far away.

Good!

Your head near your knee and then far away. What other parts of your body can you move far and near from each other?

Your knee to your nose? Who can do that? Great!

What other parts can you move near and far from each other?
Dance your hands and arms near and far from different parts of your body.

Near and far.

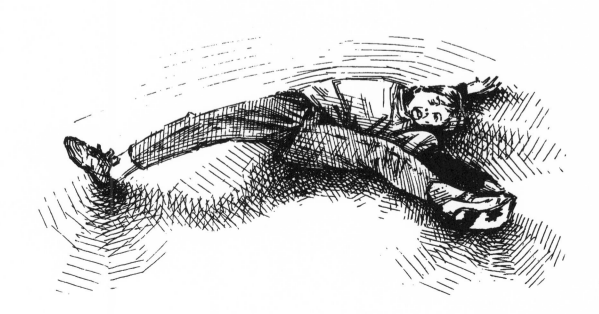

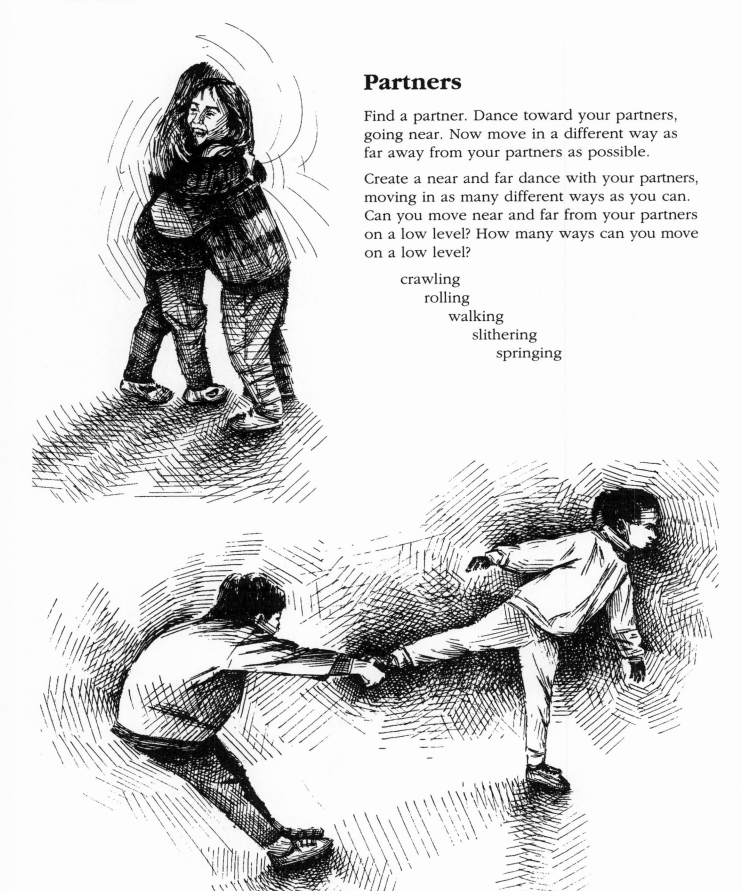

Partners

Find a partner. Dance toward your partners, going near. Now move in a different way as far away from your partners as possible.

Create a near and far dance with your partners, moving in as many different ways as you can. Can you move near and far from your partners on a low level? How many ways can you move on a low level?

crawling
    rolling
        walking
            slithering
                springing

The Star

Now you will create your own sculpture in your own space. The star (a selected student) will move in her own special way, near and far from all of the sculptures.

Watch how the star finds different ways to move near and far from each person.

Ropes

Two children will hold a long rope at each end, keeping the rope taut. Move hand over hand getting nearer and nearer to each other. You are now close enough for your hands to touch. Let the rope slide through your hands moving farther and farther away from each other.

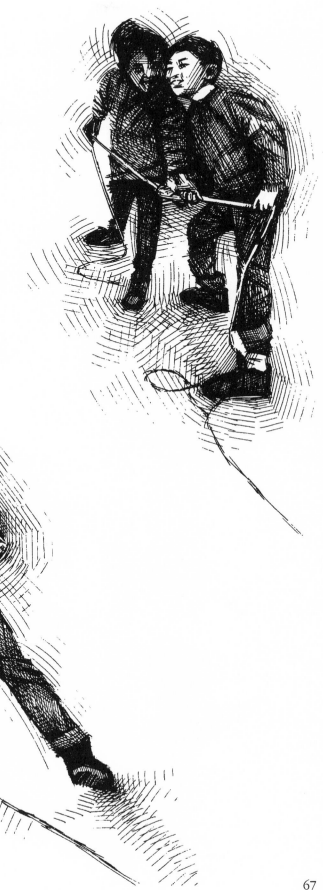

Shadow Play

With shadows, play with the idea of near and far by using your hands and feet to come closer and farther away from each other.

Awareness

Partners, stand at a distance facing each other.

One of you will move toward the other, very slowly.

Person standing still, be aware of how comfortable you are as your partner gets closer.

Tell your partner to stop as soon as you feel uncomfortable. See how much space there is between you.

Now change roles.

Move away from each other again. Then change roles. The partner who stood still will move very slowly toward the other partner.

Do you see any difference in the space each of you needs?

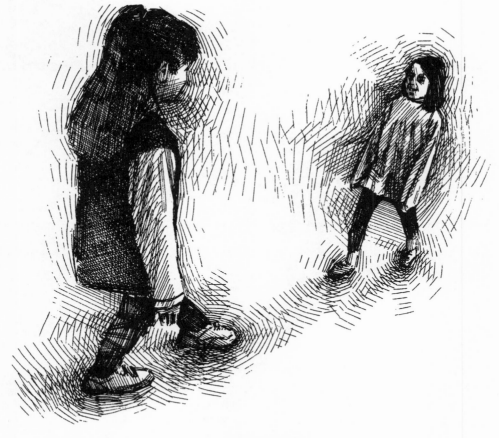

Discussion

Some of you will need more space than others between you and someone else. Talk to your partners about how much space you need to be comfortable and when you began to feel uncomfortable.

Group Dance

Dance throughout the room, meeting and parting from each other.

Dance throughout the room, meeting and then passing each other.

Now as you meet, dance together and then leave.

Continue this dance, meeting, dancing together and parting from as many partners as our dance time allows.

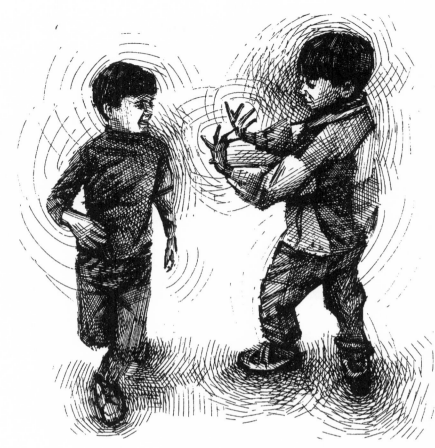

Feelings

You may all walk around in the space. As soon as you come face-to-face with someone, quickly move away. Be aware of how it feels to move away and how it feels to have that person move away from you.

Now as you move through the space and come face-to-face with someone, give that person a non-verbal greeting. Be aware of how it feels to greet someone and be greeted.

For Children with Special Needs

One person will aim her flashlight far away from herself. The rest of the children will move over to the space where the light is.

by Louise Kelsey

Can you put your hand in the light?

How about your foot?

Can you put just your head into the light?

How about your elbow?

Very good.

Now another child will have a turn shining the light, either near or far away.

By using colored lights you can extend the lesson to include colors.

Put a part of your body into that red light.

Can you put your elbow into the green light?

OVER AND UNDER

Body Parts

Can you put your hands over your head?
> Now can you put them under your chin?

Over your shoulders?
> Under your shoulders?

Over your knees?
> Under your knees?

Over your feet?
> Under your feet?

What other parts of your body can you put your hands over and under?

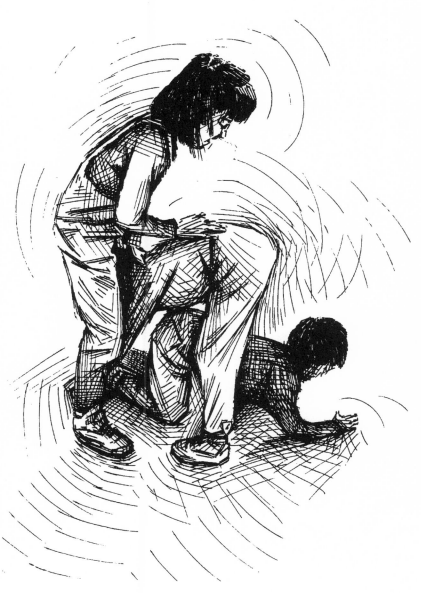

Partners

Turn toward a partner.

Place your hands over each other's shoulders.

Under each other's shoulders.

Place your leg over your partner's leg.

Under your partner's leg.

Place your _____

over your partner's_____.

Under your partner's_____.

What other parts of your body can you place over and under each other?

Experiment for a while. Then take turns showing us under and over.

Groups

How many ways can you show us under and over?

Group Dance Improvisation

Let's do an under and over dance. Move through the room slowly, and every time you come to a new person you may wave your arms or another part of your body over or under that person. You may slide under someone's legs, low down near the floor or be as tall as you can, waving your arms over that person's head and shoulders.

Experiment, using different levels and different parts of your body to go under and over each other.

Make bridges and tunnels for the others to go over or under.

Make it a dance.

Glide from one person to another,
smoothly and gracefully,
without touching. Keep finding new
ways to go over and under.

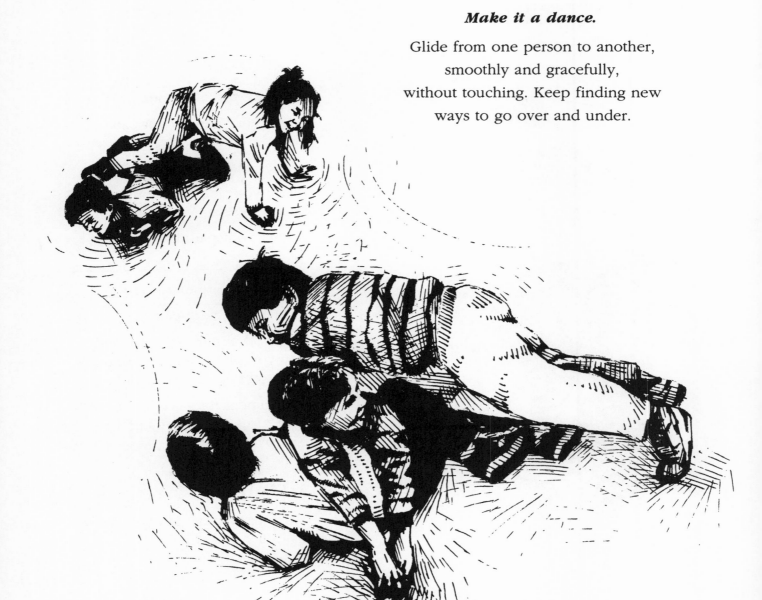

Art

Weaving Placemats

Choose two colors for the paper strips that go with the time of year. For example, red and white for Valentine's day, orange and black for Halloween, brown and orange for fall, or pastels for spring.

Collage

How many ways can you think of to paste your colored strips of paper under and over each other?

Use your imagination to make your under and over picture.

Games

Twister

Let's all hold hands in a circle except for two children not holding hands. At the break, a leader will snake us around, going over and under the arms of different people with the rest following. We do this until we are all twisted up. Then we unwind ourselves by going the opposite way.

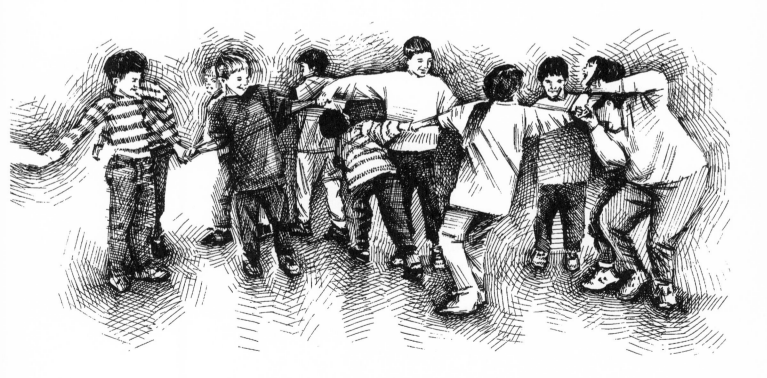

Leap Frog

Half the children will place themselves around the room. Of these, every other child will be standing with legs spread apart. The others will kneel on the floor with their heads down. The rest of us will take turns jumping over one and crawling under the next. Over and under, around we will go. Then we will change roles.

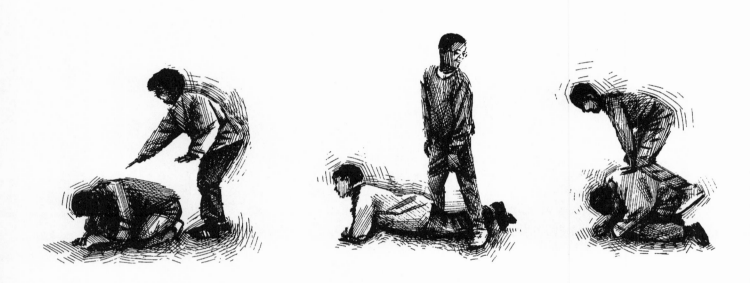

The Obstacle Course

Place furniture around the room so that children can take turns going over and under it. They can go under a table and over a yardstick placed between two chairs. Children will say "under" or "over" as they move under and over the different objects.

For Children with Special Needs

Find every opportunity to help children do motor problem solving. When you set up an activity, put up a barrier. For example, when they are used to coming into the front door you may put a bean bag in the way so that they can solve how to get around or over it in order to get into the room. These obstacles increase organizational planning. by Louise Kelsey

Pretzel

Let's do the pretzel. Stand in a circle. Give one hand to someone and the other hand to someone else. Do not give your hands to people standing next to you, and do not give both of your hands to the same person. Now, without letting go, we will try to make our circle whole again. It might end up being one large circle the way we began, two smaller circles not connected to each other, or two smaller connected circles. Let's explore how to do this. You will have to cooperate with one another, going over and under one another's arms to see whether you can untwist this pretzel.

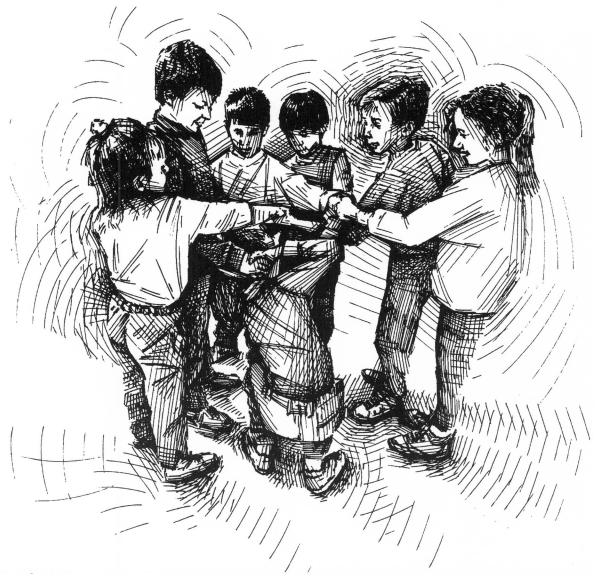

For four-year-olds, use only four children. Older children can use more in a group, but do not exceed ten.

Rope

Now we'll play the limbo game. Everyone stand in a line to go under the rope. Each time we will put the rope a little lower. Try to go under the rope without letting it touch you.

A little lower now. Great!

Now let's take turns jumping over the rope. Each time we will raise the rope a little higher. Can you jump over the rope without touching it?

Let's see how high you can jump.

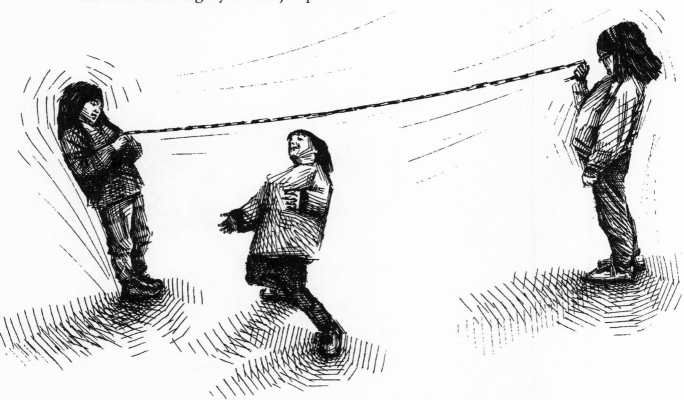

Volleyball for Children with Special Needs

We will tie a rope across two chairs. You may sit on either side facing one another. You may then throw the ball over or under the rope to each other as we say "under" or "over."

Balls

Form a line. The first person will pass the ball between his legs. The next person will receive the ball and pass it over her head. Continue passing the ball alternately under legs and over heads until it gets to the back of the line. The last person will run to the front of the line to begin again. How fast can you do this without losing the ball?

Stand in a circle. Explore sending the ball to each other using various under and over motions.

Parachute Play

donated by Chime Time

We will all hold the edge of the parachute, lifting it high and then allowing it to come down. When I call the name of a color you are wearing, run under the parachute as quickly as possible while it is still up in the air. Try to get to the other side before it comes down. Be careful not to bump into each other while you are running.

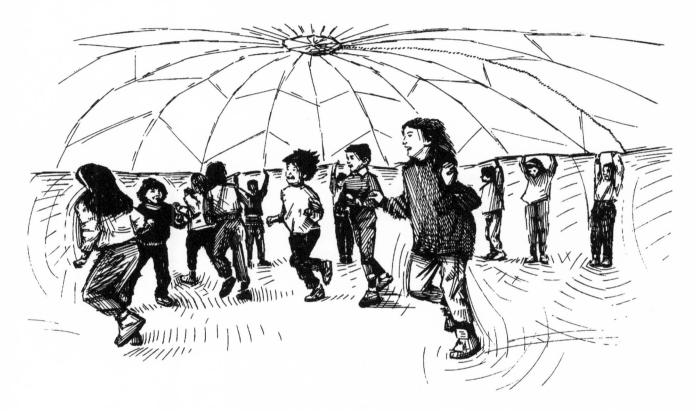

For Children with Special Needs

We will all hold on to the edge of the parachute, pulling back to make it tight. One at a time, you can make believe that you are swimming under the parachute while the rest of us try to make waves by bringing the parachute up and down.

Let's try this with more than one swimmer at a time.

This is a good way for tactile-defensive children to get used to being near each other. by Louise Kelsey

How about crawling or rolling over or under the parachute?
What are some other ways that we can move over and under the parachute?

Let's all sit down around the parachute and pull it over our legs. Where are our legs? Under the parachute. That's right!

While we are sitting here we can place our hands and arms over the parachute. What other parts of our bodies can we place over or under the parachute?

NEGATIVE AND POSITIVE

Using tubular material or Bodysox, experiment in making numerous shapes with your body. Stretch in different directions and levels. Try standing, sitting or lying down. Try stretching up high or to the sides. Experiment with curling your body and stretching it out, each time creating a different shape. We will be looking at all the interesting shapes you are making.

Now I would like you to connect to each other in your own shapes. Some of you will be standing, and some sitting or lying down. All of you will be on different levels, creating different shapes, facing in different directions and connected by some part of your body to one another.

Now I would like some of you who are not in the Bodysox to walk around and through the shapes, exploring the spaces and forms you see. Find a place that your body will fit into. Each person's sculpture is filling up positive space. The empty spaces that are created by each sculpture connected to each other are called negative space. You will find a special negative space to fit yourself into.

You may want to give your sculpture a name.

Also see "Positive and Negative Space" in *A Moving Experience*
Bodysox donated by Chime Time.

Using your stretch material, three-quarters of the class may create all kinds of different shapes while the rest may watch. Keep changing and experiment a while. Now try to connect with each other making a large sculpture and freeze in a comfortable position so that you can hold it for a while.

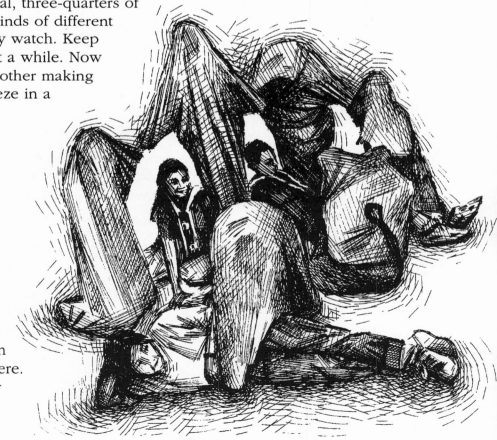

The children who are watching may walk around noticing the different shapes. You may say what you see and what it reminds you of. Now find a space to crawl in and around or fit your body into.

Find your special place in the sculpture and stay there. If you want to share why you like your space you can take turns doing so.

ON AND OFF

Body Parts

Can you put your hands on your head?
    Now take them off.
        Hands on your shoulders.
            Take them off.
What other parts of your body can you place hands on and take them off of?
    your stomach
        cheeks
            ankles
                legs
                    hips
                        knees
                            chest
                                toes
                                  elbows

Create a rhythm saying "hands on, hands off" with the names of body parts.

Can you put your ear on your shoulder?

    Take it off.

How about your elbow on your knee?

    Take it off.

Your head on your _____?

    Take it off.

Your _____ on your_____?

    Take it off.

What other good ideas do you have?

Partners

Find a partner.

Can you gently place your hands on each other's shoulders?
Take them off.

Softly on each other's heads? Take them off.
On each other's feet? Take them off.

On each other's arms? Take them off.
Very gently on each other's cheeks? Take them off.

Place your heads on each other's _____.
Take them off.

Place your legs on each other's _____.
Take them off.

What else can you place on and off each other?
What else can you think of?

Great job!

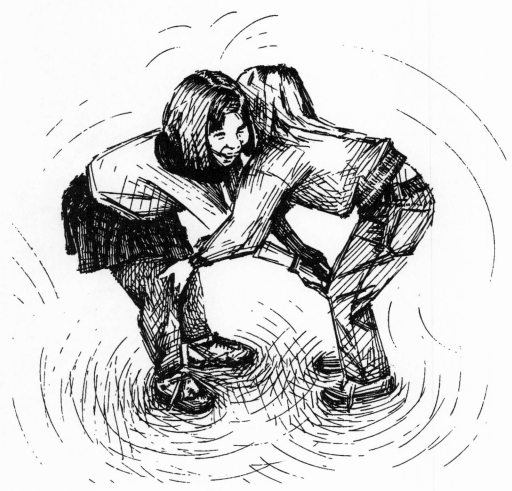

Objects

Move freely around the room, placing your hands on and off different objects while naming them.

On the table	Off the table
On the floor	Off the floor
On the chair	Off the chair
On the wall	Off the wall

What else do you see in the room to place your hands on or take them off of?

What other part of your body can you place on and take off objects?

Sit down on the chair. Now get off.

Can you put your knee on something? Take it off.

What else can you do with on and off?

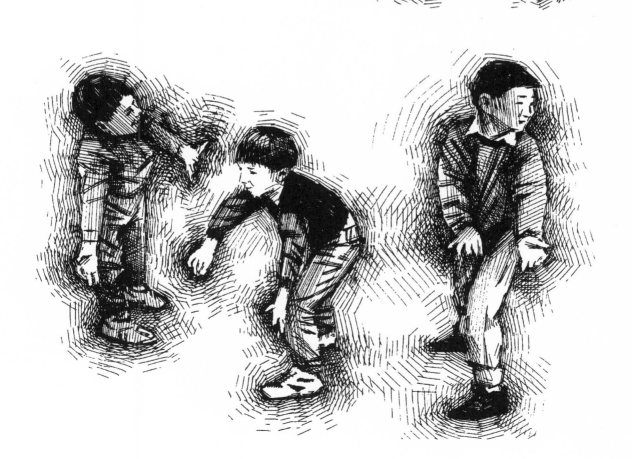

Math and Language

Place shapes on the floor around the room.

Find a shape to stand on.
    Name the shape you are on.
        Step off.
Move to another shape and step on it.
    Name the shape.
        Step off.

Continue this until interest wanes.

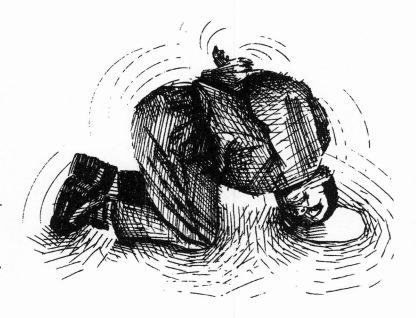

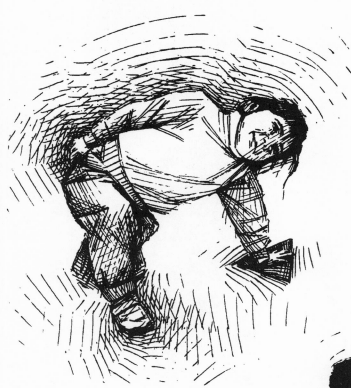

Body Parts on Shapes

Choose one shape to be on.

Place your foot on the shape. Take it off.
    Place your hand on the shape. Take it off.
      Place your elbow on the shape. Take it off.
        Place your shoulder on the shape. Take it off.

What other part of your body can
you place on and off the shape?

***You can use this activity with letters,
words, numerals or children's names.***

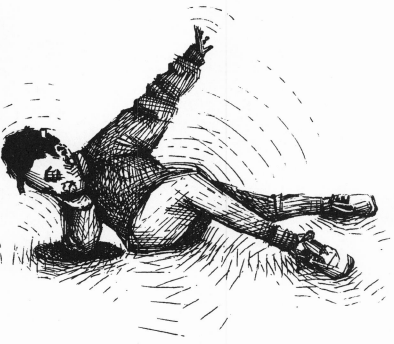

Group Dance

Play some rhythmic music.

Dance freely around the room, placing your hands on someone's back and taking them off.

Move quietly from one person to the next, placing your hands on their backs and then removing your hands. While you are touching someone's back, she can be touching someone else's arm.

Do this gently and lightly, in rhythm to the music.

Let your arms float in a dance of on and off.

What a beautiful dance!

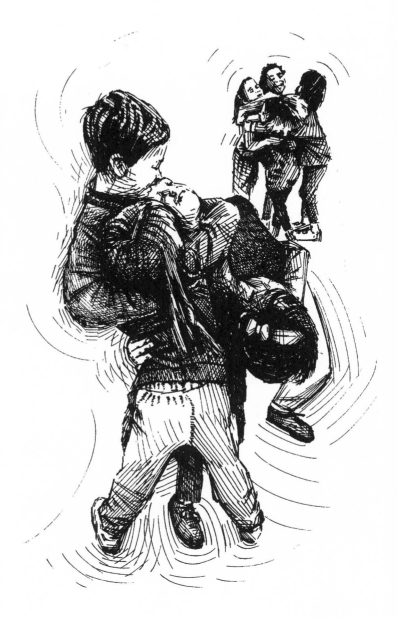

Scarves

Choose a scarf of your favorite color.

Throw it up into the air and catch it on your head.

Take it off.

Throw it up again and catch it on your elbow.

Good!

Take it off.

On what other body parts can you catch the scarf and take it off of?

Now we will do this to music, moving throughout the room, throwing the scarves into the air and catching them on different parts of our bodies, then taking them off.

Relaxation

Find a partner.

One of the partners will lie down and relax.

The partner sitting may pay attention to her breathing as another way to relax. Now you may gently place your hands on your partner's arm for a few moments. Now you may remove your hands.

Place your hands on and off your partner's

> feet,
>> shoulders,
>>> head,
>>>> arms.

Now change roles so that you all may get a turn at our on and off relaxation activity.

We can also do this in groups of three or four.

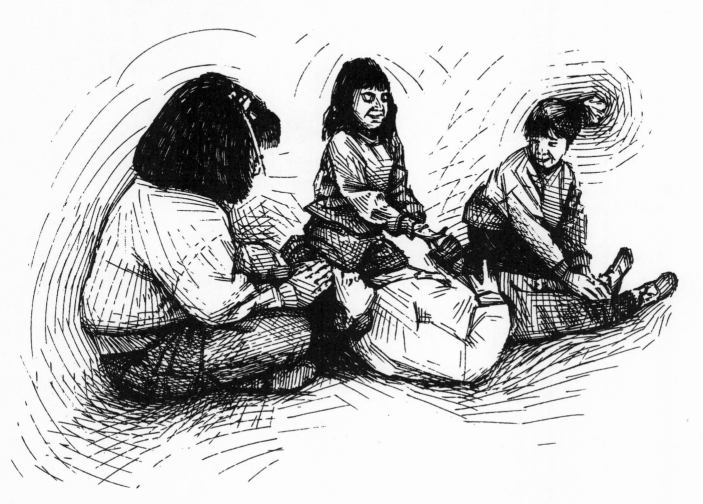

LARGE AND SMALL

Exaggerate the Movement

Everybody stand in a circle. One person will begin a movement. Now the whole group can exaggerate it, more and more and more, making the movement very large. As large as it can be.

Now we will make the movement smaller and smaller and smaller until we can hardly see it. Yes! That's great!

What kind of movements do you need to create a large dance? Possibly leaps and giant steps. What kind of movements would you use for a small dance? Possibly baby steps and little hops.

Balloons

Make believe you are a balloon that needs to be blown up. Begin by being very small and pretend someone is slowly blowing you up. The air in the balloon pushes out your arms.

Let your arms rise slowly and feel how much space your body uses.

Let's see you get **larger** and **larger** and **larger** until you are so large you think you will burst. Feel the largeness in every part of your body. Now slowly let out the air and become **smaller** and **smaller** and **smaller** until you are a tiny lump on the floor.

Sculpture

Create a very small sculpture. Now get larger and larger. Create the largest sculpture you can.

Take a partner and create a small sculpture with your partner. Now make your sculpture as large as possible.

The whole group can now make as small a sculpture as possible by one person beginning and everyone else adding on one at a time. This is your small sculpture. Now when I say "Change," you may vary the shape of your own sculpture so that it will become very large and our group sculpture will become enormous.

Space

Using as much space as possible create a large dance. How far can you reach into space? Feel the grandness of your movements. It feels so good to stretch as large as you can. Everyone may share the same space, being careful not to bump into each other and still feel your largeness and grandness.

Now begin to let your movements get smaller. Use less and less of the general space in the room. Allow your movements to become restricted to a small space. How small can your movements become? Feel your smallness. How does it feel to move in a small space and use very small movements?

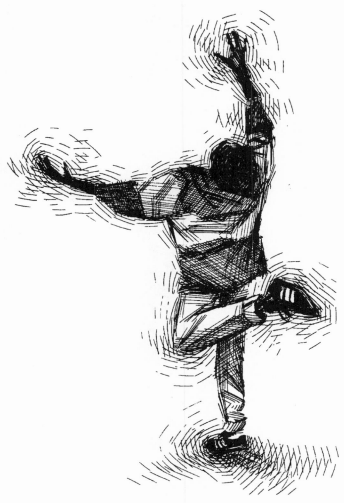

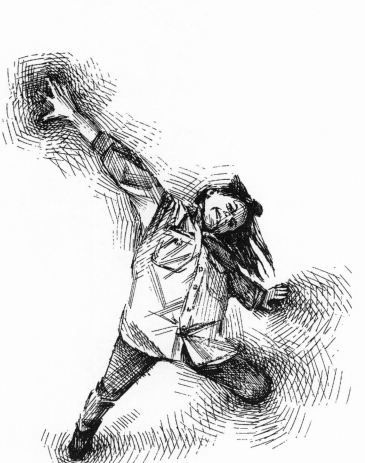

Now go back and forth between small movements in a small space and large movements in a large space and feel the difference. Use different levels with your dance. Which do you prefer? Why?

Explore the room finding all the small spaces you can fit into. Now find large spaces you can move through and around.

Animals

Which animal would you like to be to feel very large?
Hippopotamus, elephant, giraffe or lion.
Which animal would you like to be to feel very small?
Small bird, kitten, puppy, ant or mouse.
Feel that animal with your body and explore its
largeness or smallness in movement. If you chose
a small animal, now try a large one.
You may want to change from one to the other.

Shadow Play

Make larger and smaller forms by being nearer or
farther from the light source.

Parachute

Create large and small sculptures under
the parachute by adding and taking away
numbers of children.

Rope Sculpture

Place a very long rope on the floor. The
first child will pick up the end of the rope
and create a sculpture. The next child will
pick up the next part of available rope and
also create a sculpture. The next child will do
the same until the whole rope is used up and
there is a large rope sculpture. Do the same with a
smaller rope to make a small sculpture of children.

Cooperation with Large and Small

A dancer who will create large movements will begin at one end
of the room and a dancer who will create small movements
will begin at the other end of the room. Begin to dance
toward each other, slowly adjusting your movements
so that large and small will begin to be medium size
movements. Start to mirror each other, alternating
large and small movements. In this way large
and small can cooperate with each other.

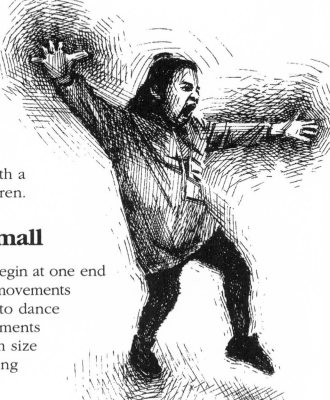

FAST AND SLOW

Body Parts

Move different parts of your body fast. How does that feel? Now move those same parts of your body slowly. How does that feel? Which do you prefer?

How many parts of your body can you find to move fast and slow?

eyes

toes

chin

fingers

hips

legs

Great! There are so many parts of our body that can move either fast or slow.

Partners

Take a partner and experience moving fast and slow with each other.

Try moving in the opposite way from each other. One of you may move very slowly while the other moves fast. Now try it the other way.

Find ways to move together very slowly while continuing to make eye contact. Allow all parts of your body to feel the slowness of your movements while you are relating to your partner in your slow dance.

Now gradually allow your movements to become faster and faster until you are doing your fast dance while still keeping control. This is a nontouching fast dance with your partner. You are still relating to each other in some way while moving as fast as you can. Now freeze!

Ribbons

Use long ribbons of various colors swirling them fast and then slow. Let's use fast music to help us move quickly and then slow music to inspire us to move slowly.

How many designs can you make with your ribbons as you move them very fast and then slowly?

Animals

Can you think of an animal that moves very fast? The fastest animal is a cheetah. How about a slow animal, such as a turtle or a snail? Let's be that kind of animal, moving either fast or slow.

Machines

What kind of machines can you think of that move either fast or slow? Let's be that machine.

What kind of machine are you? Let the rest of us guess. Try creating a machine with a partner. Does your machine run fast or slow?

Try creating a machine in small groups. Maybe some parts of the machine will be running fast while other parts need to run slowly.

Water

Let's make believe we are water. We can be a fast moving brook or a slow moving lake.

What other things can you think of that move fast or slow?

WIDE AND NARROW

Body Parts

How wide can you spread your fingers? Now make the spaces between your fingers as narrow as possible.

How wide can you spread your arms?

Your legs?

Bring your legs in to make as narrow a space between them as possible. Now do that with your arms.

How can you make yourself feel and look very wide?

Walk around the room as if you need a great deal of space for yourself.

How does it feel to be so wide?

Puff out your face. Stick out your stomach.

Now make yourself narrow, as narrow as an arrow.

You can move through the smallest spaces because you are so narrow.

Move through the room, feeling the narrowness of your body.

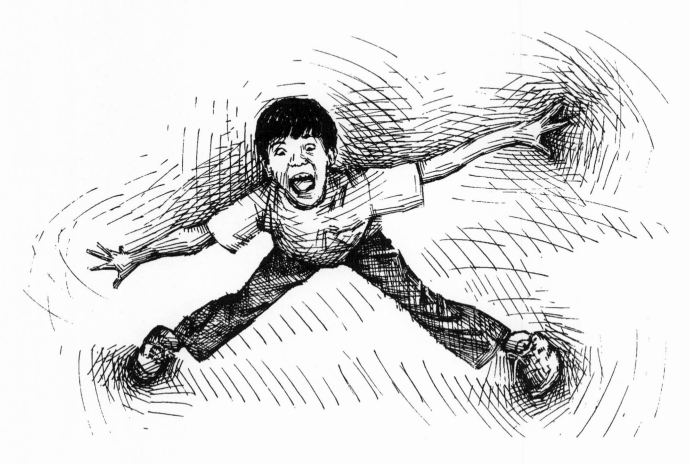

The Dance

Create a dance, being alternately as narrow and as wide as you can be as you move throughout the space. Be aware of the transition as you go from wide to narrow and narrow to wide.

Feel how stretched your body is when you are wide and how closed in and tight it feels when you are narrow.

How many ways can you show wide and narrow with your body?

Try doing this on different levels. How about being narrow and low to the floor? How about being wide and as high up as you can be?

Try different combinations of high and low and narrow and wide.

Try a wide dance with flowing movements. Try a narrow dance with sharp movements.

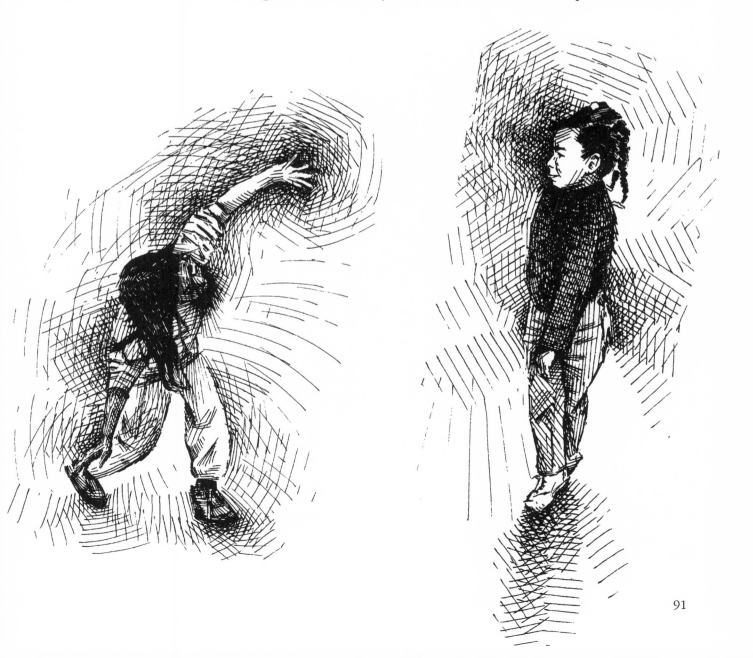

Partners

One of you will be narrow and one will be wide. Face and watch each other as you both go slowly from narrow to wide and from wide to narrow. Go back and forth for a while as if you were dancing.

Feel the narrowness or wideness in every part of your body:

> your face
>> arms
>>> chest
>>>> hips
>>>>> and legs.

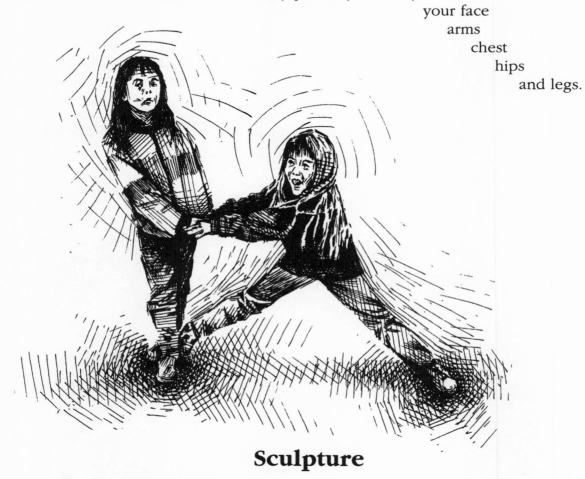

Sculpture

Create a sculpture with your partner to show wide. Now change the sculpture to show narrow.

Make a different sculpture to show wide. And a different way to show narrow.
Join another pair of partners to become a group of four.

> Create a sculpture to show narrow. Now change it to wide.
>> Now narrow.
>>> Change to wide.

Combine your group with another group of four to become a group of eight. Create a sculpture showing narrow. Change your sculpture to wide.

> Now narrow. Change to wide.
>> Narrow.
>>> Wide.

Mirroring

Now we will just be narrow. One of you will move slowly, as narrow as you can, and your partner will mirror your narrowness. Move slowly so that your partner can follow you easily.

Now change roles. The other person will be the leader and the partner will do the mirroring.

Let's do this again, this time feeling our wideness. Each partner will have a turn being the mirror and the leader.

Leader, now you will go from narrow to wide and from wide to narrow, with your mirror following you. Watch your mirror to see whether you are getting the feeling of wide and narrow.

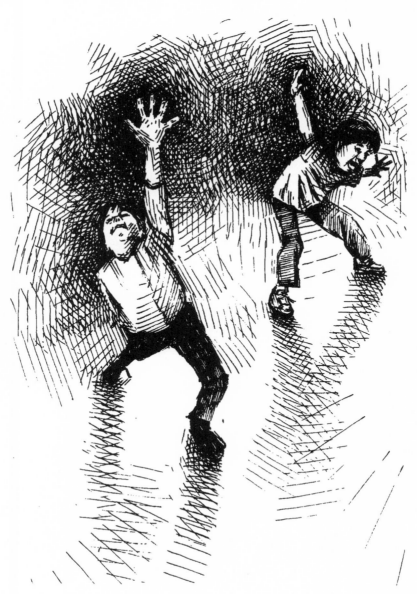

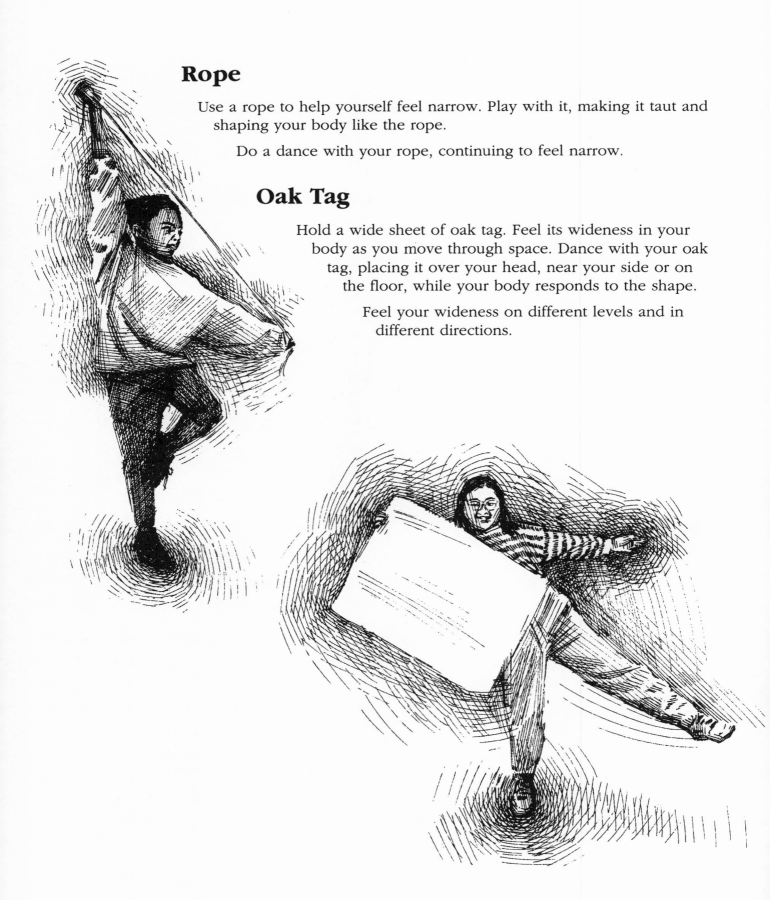

Rope

Use a rope to help yourself feel narrow. Play with it, making it taut and shaping your body like the rope.

Do a dance with your rope, continuing to feel narrow.

Oak Tag

Hold a wide sheet of oak tag. Feel its wideness in your body as you move through space. Dance with your oak tag, placing it over your head, near your side or on the floor, while your body responds to the shape.

Feel your wideness on different levels and in different directions.

Fantasy

Can you blow yourself up like a balloon and float around the room feeling wide?
Can you make yourself as narrow as sewing thread to go through the eye of a needle?

For Children with Special Needs
by Louise Kelsey

Drape fabrics over the backs of chairs to create a wide aisle.

Move down the aisle between the chairs with your arms out to the sides, letting your fingertips touch the fabrics. Feel how wide you can be.

Drape the chairs with something smooth, such as oilcloth and move the chairs closer to each other to make a narrow aisle.

Feel your narrowness as you crawl through this channel.

All children can participate in this activity. You can vary the fabrics to promote and encourage sensory awareness. Fingertips touching textured fabrics such as an afghan, flannel blankets or corduroy are good for wide; bare shoulders touching smooth fabrics are good for narrow.

Angels

Lie down on the oilcloth and make angels. See how we can make ourselves both wide and narrow as we do this.

Art

Collage

Prepare strips of narrow and wide paper in various colors.
Arrange them in a collage to create something either abstract or representational.

String Painting

Dip a piece of string into a paint jar. Now drag it across your paper creating narrow lines. Do this with various colors.

For wide, take the painted string at both ends and draw it across the paper creating wide shapes. Do this in various colors.

You may want to create a painting combining both wide and narrow shapes. Create your wide shapes first and then go over the wide dry paint with narrow lines.

You can also dip the wide side of a rectangle shaped cardboard into paint and drag it down the paper, creating wide strokes. Let's do this with the narrow side of the cardboard and create narrow strokes. It looks great!

What else can you use to create wide and narrow?

PUSH AND PULL

Pushing

Push with your arms as if you are in water up to your neck.
Feel the water resisting you.
Feel the tension in your arms.
Now lie down and push with your feet
and legs as if you were pushing a
strong wall. Feel the tension
in your legs as you do
this. Move around the
room, letting your
shoulder lead you.
Feel your shoulder
pushing as if a strong
wind were holding you back.
Now lead with your head.
Let your head lead you through
the room. The wind is quite
strong, but you can move
with strength. Now lead with your
chest. Push with all your might.

You will find that you can only move slowly against the wind.
What other body part can you push with?
Do that now.

Dance

Allow one body part to
lead and then another,
moving through the
room, pushing against
the strong wind.

Do this in slow motion.
Shift smoothly from one
part of your body to
another.

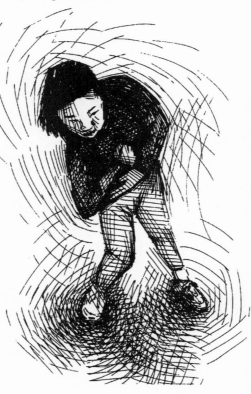

For Children with Special Needs
by Louise Kelsey

Push as hard as you
can against the walls or
other strong stationary
objects. Pretend you
are pushing out to a
larger space.

***This will give the
children a feeling
of expansion.***

Partners

Face a partner, allowing some space between you. Place the palms of your hands against each other. Begin pushing gently so that neither of you will fall. See how many different positions you can find while pushing.

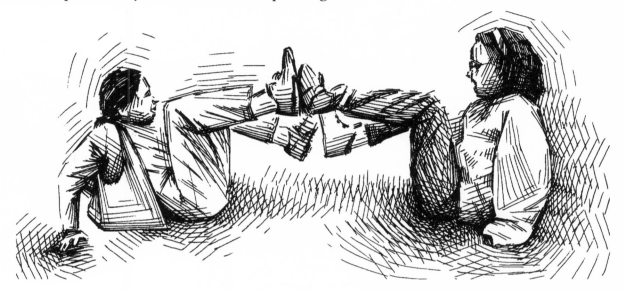

Lie down on your backs opposite your partner, with your legs in the air. Let the bottoms of your feet touch. See how many ways you can push. Push with one leg and then the other or let them both go in the same direction. Good!

You may want to sing the following to the tune of "Skip to My Lou":
Push, push, push my legs
Push, push, push my legs
Push, push, push my legs
Push my legs with my part-ner.

A child whose legs were affected by cerebral palsy enjoyed this exercise with his partner. He didn't like having his legs exercised in physical therapy, but with a peer for a partner, it was fun. While learning cooperative play and the concept of pushing, he was also doing the appropriate exercises for strengthening his legs.

Now sit back to back. Allow your backs to push against each other. Rock back and forth for a while. You may try to stand and then sit again, with the support of each other's back. Try some other ways of pushing back to back, to see what you can accomplish with the support of your partner. Try this in groups of three.

Push Dance with a Partner

Gently push each other, going from one body part to another. Experience the pressure of pushing. Use your　　　　hips　　　　　　　　legs
　　　　　　　　　　　　backs　　　　　　　　　chest
　　　　　　　　　　　　　shoulders　　　　　　　arms.

Feel the support of your partner's pushing and use that to help you move in different directions and at different levels. Do this gently and in slow motion.

Group of Four

Join another pair and make a group of four. Gently and slowly, push each other using different parts of your body. Go from one person to the next, using different directions and levels. Allow your whole body to respond to the pushing, creating new movements in your body.

Group Push

　　　Begin in a circle with everyone facing in the same direction of either right or left. Push on each other's backs while everyone leans slightly backward.
　　　Face toward the center of the circle with hands facing and pressing those on either side of you.
　　　What other types of group pushing can you do?
Let different parts of your body push each other gently and slowly while those being
　　　pushed resist the push by pushing back gently.

For Children with Special Needs

Through movement I am sometimes able to change acting out into an appropriate behavior. For example, one day when I was demonstrating a pushing exercise in a special education class, a child aggressively pushed another while they were playing.

Oh, you are pushing. Let's sit you back to back (*as I maneuvered them*) and do the "pushing game." Good pushing! You are doing a great job!

The children were smiling and enjoying each other as they pushed, and the child who thought he was going to be punished for acting out felt validated and good about himself. I arranged the other children back to back with a partner of equal size and strength so that they were all able to participate in this new pushing experience.

Timmy, who was tactile-defensive, seemed able to tolerate back to back contact. By expanding the push-pull lesson we met the needs of one more child.

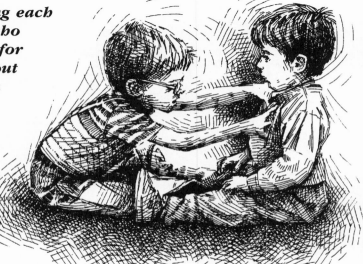

Balls

Push extra huge balls around the room. You may bounce on them, roll on them and push them with different parts of your body.

Play a game with others, pushing the ball back and forth, always using a different part of your body.

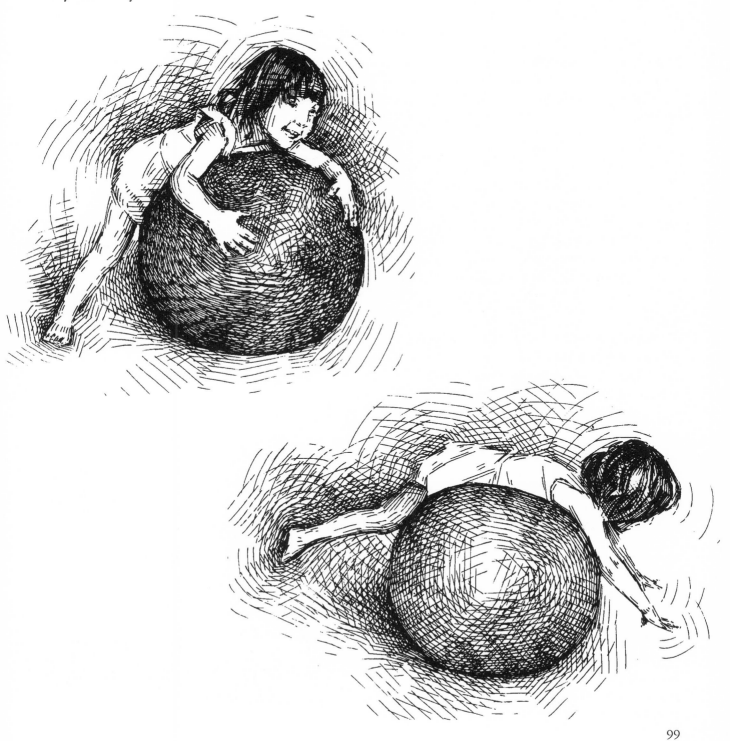

Pulling

Partners

Find a partner. Take each other's wrists and pull gently. See how many different positions you can get into while pulling. Make believe you are rubber bands, stretching yourselves as you pull.

Try this holding only one wrist.

Pulling Dance

Take your partner's hand. Take turns pulling each other gently and slowly around the room, creating different shapes and patterns as you move.

Use the whole space.
   Sometimes you might pull your partner toward you.

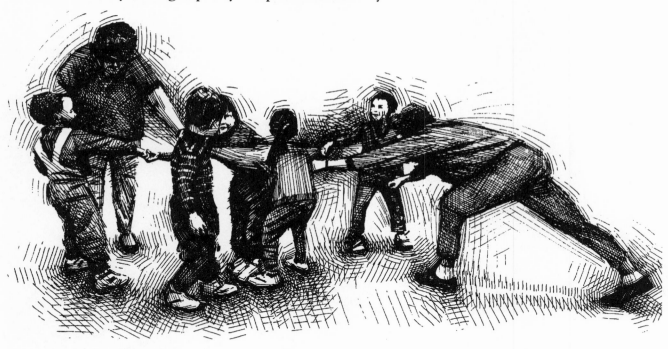

The one pulling creates a dance with her partner's body. The one being pulled allows his body to respond in different ways. See how many shapes your body moves into while you are being pulled.

Ropes

Holding a rope between yourself and your partner, pull in different directions. See all of the shapes you can create!

Try this with a stretch rope.

Threesome

Hold the hands of two people on either side of you. Gently pull, creating different movements while your partners support you.

Group

Make a large circle, with all holding the wrists of those next to you. Now pull each other gently. Some of you may bend your legs and slowly move down as you are being pulled. Others may be moving toward the center of the circle and others may be moving backward.

See how many different positions you can take and how differently the circle can be shaped as you gently pull on the wrists of those on both sides of you.

One designated person may drop the wrist of the person on one side of her. Now let the circle move in different directions as you all pull. Some of you may be on the floor, still pulling very slowly.

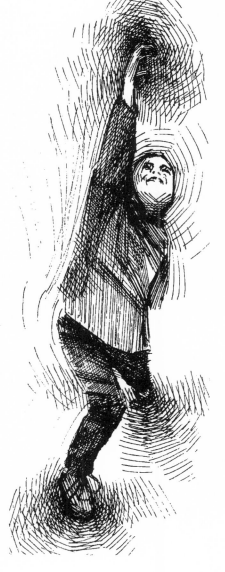

Fantasy

Make believe a string attached to your elbow is pulling you around the room. Now the string is attached to your head. It continues to pull you around the room.

What other body part can the string be attached to?
Your shoulder. Good!
Your hip, your fingers! Good!

Let's see you move through the space as if a string were pulling that part of your body.

What other parts can the imaginary string pull?
Your chin,
nose,
ear,
heels,
back? Great!

Now create a dance, shifting the string to different parts of your body. We will be able to tell where the string is pulling you by your movements. Don't forget to let that part lead while the rest of your body follows.

Try being pulled fast or slow, straight, zigzag or in circles, smoothly or bumpily. How else can the string pull you?

Dance Improvisation

Using as many parts of your body as you can, pull toward you all the things you like. Gather in all you desire. Take it in from the sky and let it flow through you, down your arms and down your body. Do this in rhythm as in a dance. Tell us what you are pulling toward you. Now using pushing movements, push away all things you do not want and everything that is negative to you. Push them far away. Push with your feet, hands and shoulders. Push them away with all your might.

Now alternate with push and pull. Do your push and pull dance using your whole body and all the space. Take what you want and get rid of what you don't want.

Yes! That's the way. It's a beautiful dance.

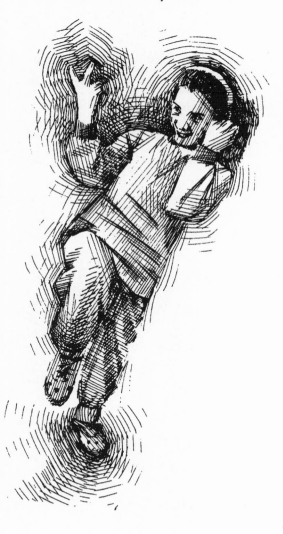

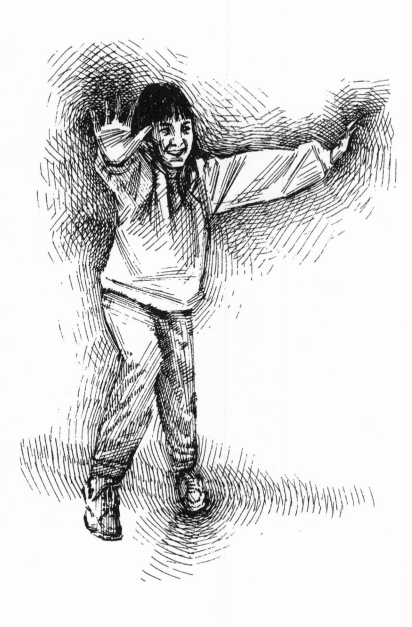

TIGHT AND LOOSE

Relaxation

Find a space that is not near anyone else
    and lie down on your back.
Tighten your fists as hard as you can.
    Tighter, tighter, tighter!
And let go completely.
    Now tighten your whole arm.
Tighter, tighter, tighter!
    Good! Now let go completely.

We will do this with all parts of your body.
    face and neck,   hips,
      shoulders,   legs,
        stomach,   back,
          feet and toes,
whole body very tight,
    and let go, feeling loose.
      Take a deep breath in and let go.

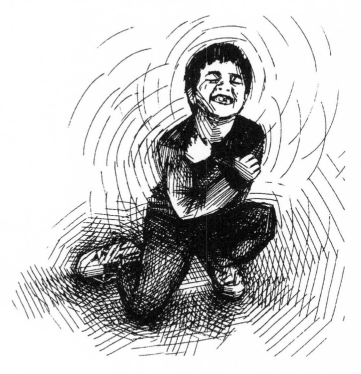

Dancing

Can you dance like a rag doll and
    be all loose and wobbly?
How many ways can you move as
    a loose wobbly rag doll?
Can you be a tin soldier and create
    a stiff tight dance?
How many ways can you move
    stiffly as a tight tin soldier?
Let's go back and forth between
    tight and loose.
Be aware of which you like better,
    a tight or a loose dance.

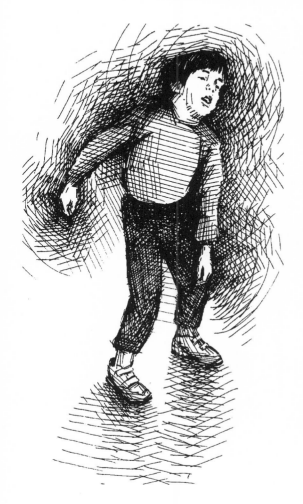

Discussion

Which did you like better, tight or loose? Why?

For the Child with Special Needs
by Louise Kelsey

Exaggerate movement so that children can experience the sensations more deeply. It helps to pair the activity with language.

UP AND DOWN
HIGH AND LOW
OR RISE AND SINK

Body Parts

Look up to the sky and now down to the earth.

Point your nose up to the sky and now down to the earth.

Stick your tongue up to the sky and now down to the earth.

What other part of your body can you move up and down?

Your fingers! *Good!*

What other part of your body can you move up and then down?

Your arms!

Yes! Let's use our arms.

Continue asking for more parts of the body that can go up and down. Use whatever the children suggest. If you don't know how to make your stomach go up and down, ask the child for a demonstration.

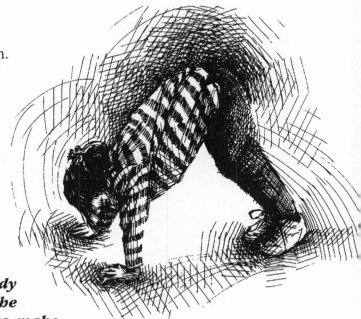

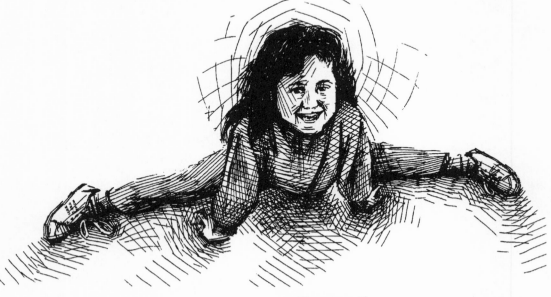

Sound

On the piano or xylophone I will play notes going up and down. Try moving on the same level you are hearing. Listen to the changes. Use your arms and whole body, allowing the movement to flow from one to another to create a dance of up and down.

You may also listen and respond to how fast or slow I am playing.

Partners

Take a partner and create a series of up-and-down movements together. You may both go up and then down or you may alternate. Try going up and down while holding hands or leaning against each other's backs.

Create a dance in which you are going up and down throughout the room.

Show us the dance.

Okay, let's watch half the couples do their up-and-down dance while the rest of us appreciate you. Then we will switch so we can enjoy the other dancers.

Whole Group

Move through the room, going up and down in as many different ways as you can think of.

Find your own way to move high up toward the sky and then down low toward the earth.

Make it your own dance.

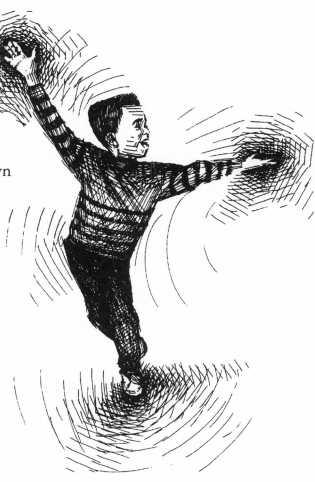

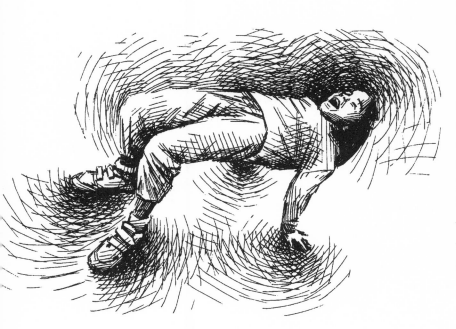

Be careful not to bump into anyone else.

Stand in a circle and count off—
one, two, one, two—
all the way around.

When I say "Go," all of the ones will bend down and the twos will rise up on their toes and change direction. Every other person will be going up while the others are going down.

What other kinds of games can we invent for going up and down?

Parachute
donated by Chime Time

Everyone bend down, and together we will lift the parachute as high as we can. Then take three steps toward the center to make a balloon. Then let the parachute fall gently by itself. Let's do it again. Up and down.

Hold the parachute with one hand, everyone facing in the same direction. Walk around as if you are on a merry-go-round, bending up and down with the parachute. Let's march in rhythm going up and down. Now let's jazz it up, still going up and down.

Make huge waves with the parachute by making it go up and down. Now let's put a lot of balls on top of the parachute. When we shake the parachute up and down, the balls will also bounce up and down. Have fun and experiment by trying to keep all the balls on top of the parachute.

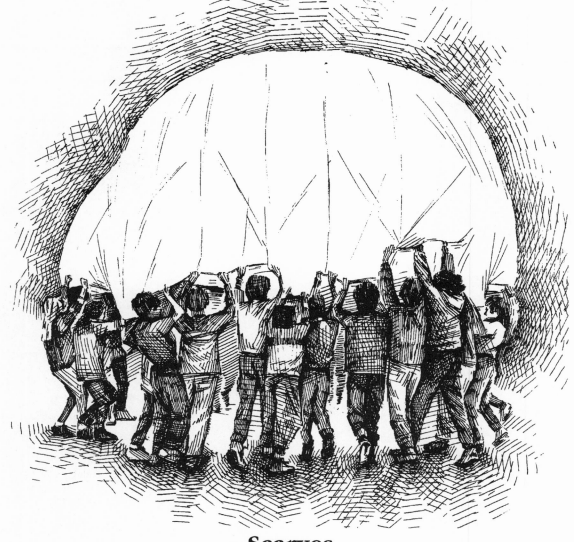

Scarves

Throw scarves up in the air and watch them come down, landing on different parts of your body.

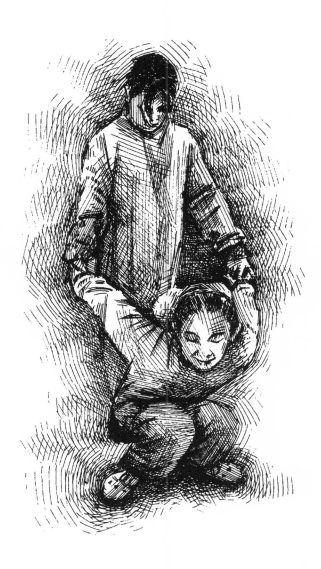

See-Saw

How about going up and down on a
see-saw? We can make believe we are on a
see-saw by holding hands with a partner.
One will go down while the other one is
up and then the reverse. Up and down we
go with our partner on the see-saw.

How many different ways can you create a
see-saw with your partner?
Try this using different directions.
Try different levels.

Passive/Active

Find a partner. One of you will
manipulate your partner's arms
and legs making them go up and
down in different shapes. Make
sure your partner is sitting when
you shape his or her legs to go
up and down.

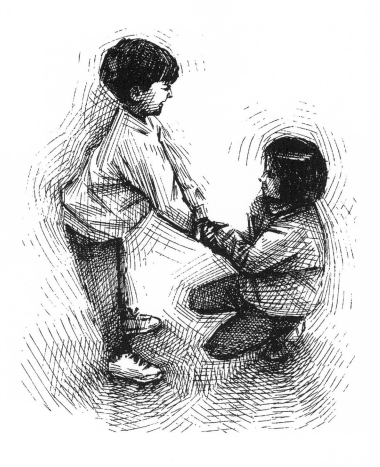

Human Up and Down Trust Exercise

A group of about twenty children stand ten in a row, facing each other, holding on to each other's arms at the shoulders. They form a strong nest for our trust exercise. Another person lies face down into their arms. The children bounce him up and down in a forward direction. Our trusting person moves slowly through the nest as the children gently bounce him up and down. Someone at the other end will help lift him off.

Thank you Ron Roberts for your idea

For Children with Special Needs

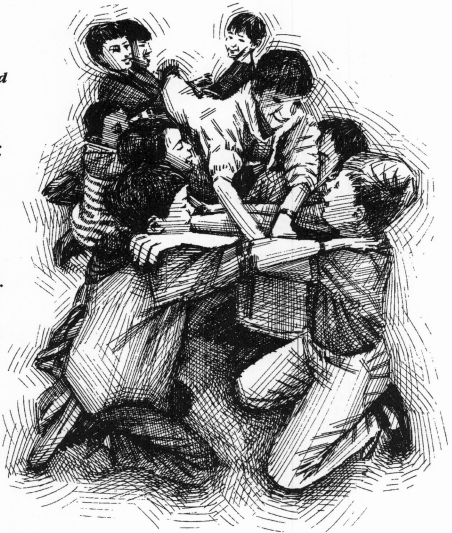

Bob, a gentle four-year-old boy with cerebral palsy, was encouraged to move a four-year-old girl who could not support herself.

He took her fragile hand and slowly moved it up and down. Both children were concentrating on the movement of her hand. She was smiling at the gentle attention of her new friend.

Here was an opportunity for a child who could not move herself to be meaningfully manipulated in an enjoyable way by a child who was more physically mobile and sociable.

One child was learning new ways in which her body could move, and the active sculptor could see the immediate result of his thoughtfulness and creativity. Both were learning to participate in a creative relationship, experiencing gentle touch and responsibility for one another.

ENDING AND BEGINNING

Changes

One at a time, come into the center and become a sculpture by attaching to one another. You will be attached with different body parts. Be on different levels and create different shapes, but maintain a line formation. The line does not have to be straight. It could curve in different ways.

After all of you are in the sculpture, the first person may move to the back of the line, attach in a different way and create a new shape.

Be aware of each other so that only one person at a time is moving.

> Let's do it faster.
> Now let's do it in slow motion.
> Keep this going.
> You may want to change the direction of the line.

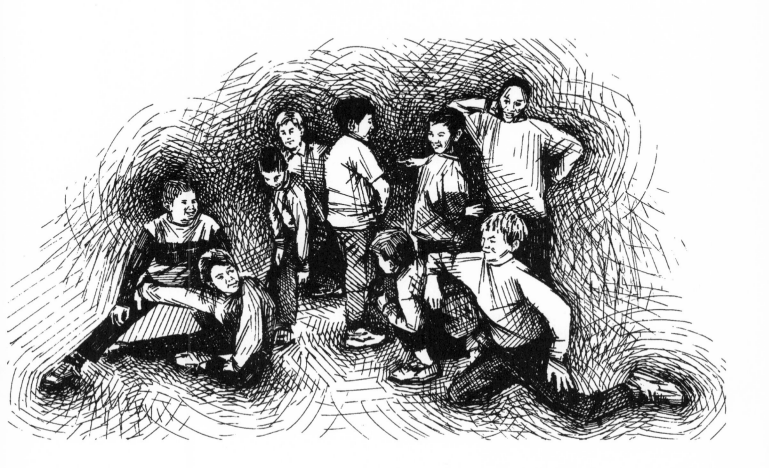

LIGHT AND HEAVY

Fantasy

Lie down and close your eyes. Take three deep breaths. I will count to six as you inhale. Hold your breath to the count of three and exhale slowly to the count of six. Ready!

Now imagine you are lying down on a white fluffy cloud. You are very relaxed and the cloud is beginning to float up slowly through a beautiful clear blue sky. Feel your lightness as you float. Feel the softness of the cloud as you are floating. Feel your body giving in to the softness and how good it feels. Feel the spaciousness of the sky. Allow yourself to feel that spaciousness. There is a gentle breeze blowing your cloud and taking you on a slow, gentle ride. Let the cloud take you to a special joyful place of your own choosing. Describe the place to yourself and what you would like to do there. I will be silent for a few moments while you enjoy your journey, feeling light while floating on your gentle airy cloud.

Now I would like you to begin to feel a little heavier. Slowly the wind is bringing you and your cloud down to earth. Sinking, sinking very slowly as the cloud lights upon the floor and you are now experiencing a sinking feeling. Feel yourself getting heavier and heavier and let yourself give in to the floor. Feel yourself letting go and getting heavier. Feel the floor beneath your body and how it feels as you grow heavier.

Slowly you may begin to move. First move your fingers and toes. Lazily allow your arms and legs to move. Stretch your entire body. Be aware of the room you are in and all the other people. Slowly open your eyes and when you are ready you may sit up in a relaxed position.

Movement

Stand with your feet planted firmly on the floor. Let yourself feel very heavy. Slowly allow your shoulders to feel their heaviness and begin to bring your body down. Slowly your head drops and your whole body sinks to the floor. Feel your heaviness.

Now you will begin to feel lighter and lighter. As you are feeling lighter and lighter, you will find yourself rising until you are fully standing. You may be feeling so light you'll want to stand on your toes.

Now begin to let the lightness move you through the space. Maybe you can be a balloon or a feather moving lightly through the room. How would a feather move? Let your arms and legs feel the lightness. Do your light dance. You can make believe you are a puppet with someone pulling the strings. Let your body move through the room as a puppet without gravity, bouncing and springing through the space.

Now move through the room feeling heavy. Pretend to push a large piano. Push the piano with different parts of your body. Try moving through the room on different levels, letting different parts of your body lead. Feel the heaviness as you move. Feel how much energy it takes to move such a heavy body.

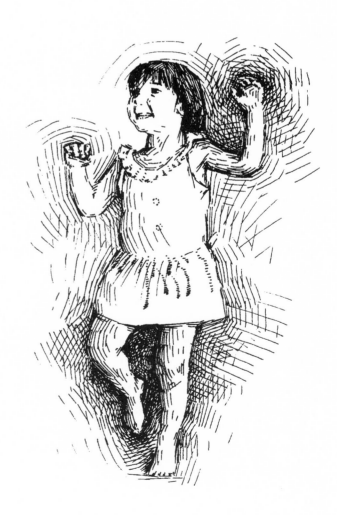

Feel as if you are a pendulum. Swing your arms from side to side and each time you swing down, feel the heaviness of the movement. This gives you momentum as you swing.

Now we will go back and forth between light and heavy. Fall to the floor like a ton of bricks and feel your heaviness as you lie there. Now slowly rise as if you were a leaf picked up by the wind.

Create a light and heavy dance going from one to the other.

How many ways
    can you feel your lightness?
       How many ways
           can you feel your heaviness?

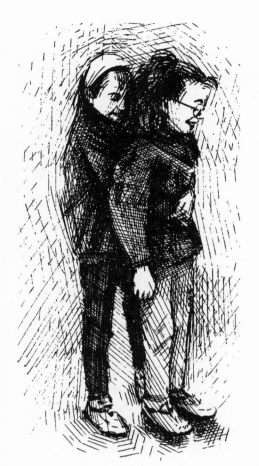

Partners

Stand one behind the other facing in the same direction. I would like you to make yourself feel as heavy as possible. Think heavy. Feel your feet planted on the floor as if they have glue on them. Feel as if you are sinking down while still standing. All parts of your body feel as if your weight is going down into the floor, feeling very heavy.

Standing behind your partner, gently put your arms around your partner's waist and try lifting her. You don't have to actually lift her or him off the floor. Just get a feeling of your partner's weight. Be careful so that you or your partner don't fall. This is not a competition.

Okay, you may now step back from your partner. Partner in front, I would like you to feel very light. Feel as if a wind can pick you up and blow you away.

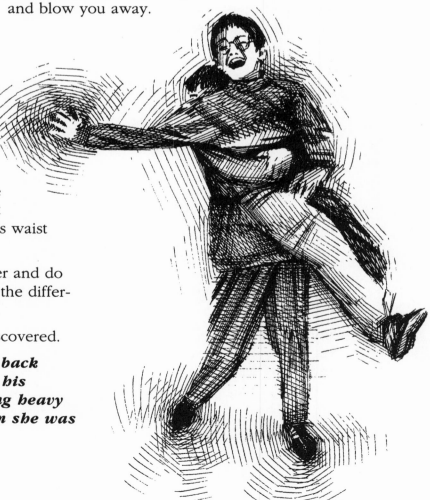

Think up as if you are floating higher and higher and higher. All your energy is going up. Now partner in the back, you may again gently put your arms around your partner's waist and try lifting her or him.

Change places with your partner and do this again so you can both feel the differences between light and heavy.

Let's talk about what you've discovered.

In most cases the person in back found it very difficult to lift his partner when she was feeling heavy but it was much easier when she was feeling light.

STRONG AND GENTLE

Drum Beats

Listen to the drum beats and respond to strong or light sounds.

What kinds of movements will you create to light drum beats? An easy walk or tip toe? Let your whole body respond to the light beats. Find all the ways you can move lightly.

Now listen to the strong beats and let your body respond to strength. What kinds of movements will you use to show strength?

Jumping or stamping with lots of energy.
What other parts of your body can you use to show strength?
Let's put light and strong together to make a dance.
Listen to the drum beats and respond with strong
or light movement, going from one to another.
Let your whole body be involved in response
to light and strong sounds.

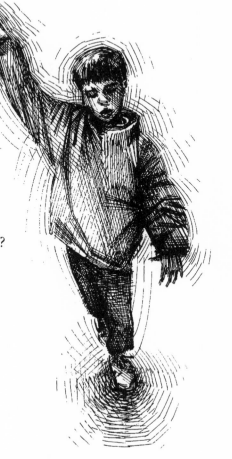

Cooperation with Strong and Gentle

One person who will dance with strong
movements and another who will dance with gentle
movements begin at opposite sides of the room.

Finding all the possible ways you can move, create your gentle
and strong dance.

Now as you begin to come toward the center, change your
movements so that they will be similar when you meet.
Begin to mirror each other experiencing both strong and
gentle movements.

How did it feel to adjust your movements to another's?

IN AND OUT

Individual Body Parts

Put one hand on your hip to create a space. Put the other arm in and then take it out.

Put your feet together and bend your knees, creating a space between your legs. Place your hand, arm, elbow in and then take it out, of that space.

Is there another way you can create a space with one part of your body and then place another part in and out of it?

Partners

It is easier to do this with a partner. One partner will make a shape and the other will go in and out of that shape. One of you can be a bending tree and the other an animal that is trying to get shelter by being close.

Now come out.

Hoops

Place different parts of your body in and out of your hoop. Let's do this in rhythm naming the body part and saying "in" and "out."

My foot goes in and out of the circle.

My elbow goes in and out of the circle.

Choose a partner to work with.

Our bottoms go in and out of the circle.

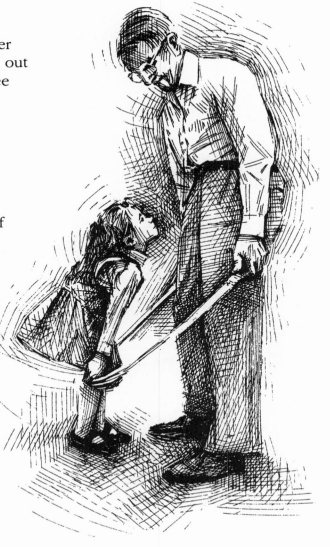

Dance

Do a jumping in and out dance as you say "in" and "out."

Each time you jump in and out do it a different way.

Use your whole body in this dance of in and out.

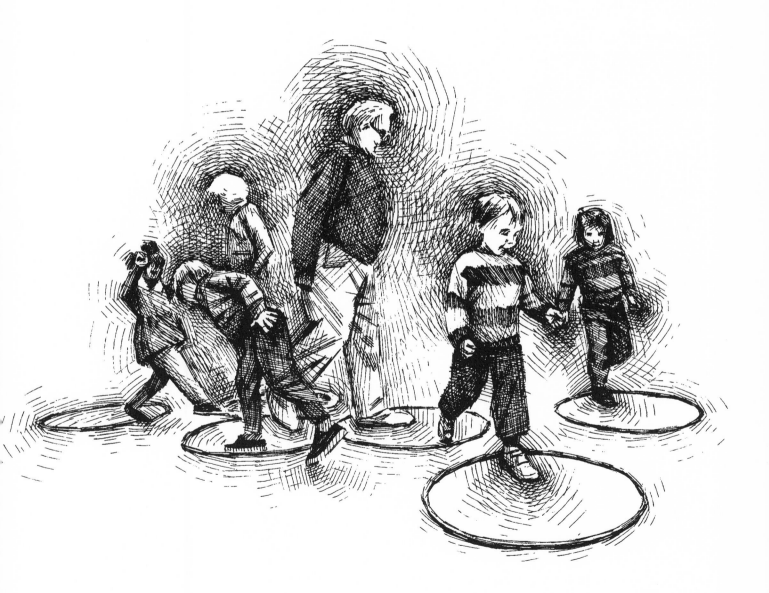

Games

Squirrel In the Tree

Two or three children create a circle with one child who is the squirrel inside, making many circles to involve all children. There will be one extra child who doesn't have a tree. When a signal is given, all the children in the centers of the circles run out of their trees and find different trees. This will give the extra child a chance to also find a tree. There will always be one child left who is not in a tree. They are the Queen or King of Squirrels.

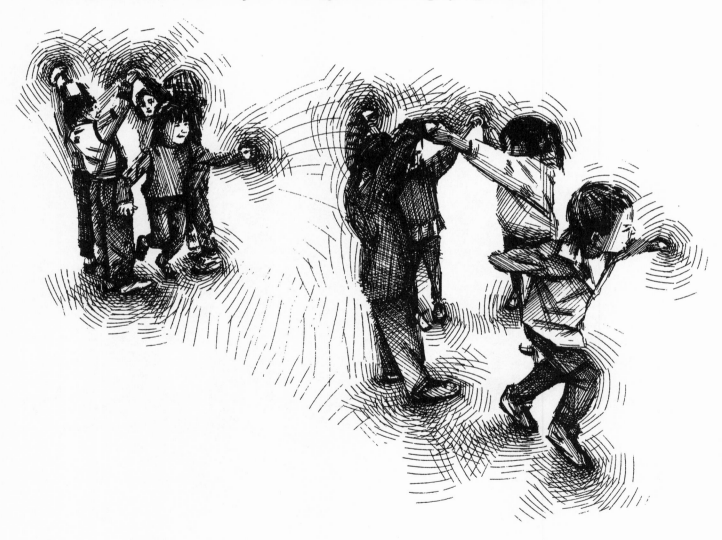

This does not have to be done competitively. It is a lot of fun and it is also fun to be the extra. It is a matter of how the child in the center is treated. The signal is given quickly so that the child in center is not there very long.

Bluebird

Song

Bluebird, bluebird, through my window,
Bluebird, bluebird through my window,
Bluebird, bluebird through my window,
Oh, (child's name), I am tired.
Take a little child and tap her on the shoulder,
Take a little child and tap her on the shoulder,
Take a little child and tap her on the shoulder,
Oh, (child's name), I am tired.
Start again.

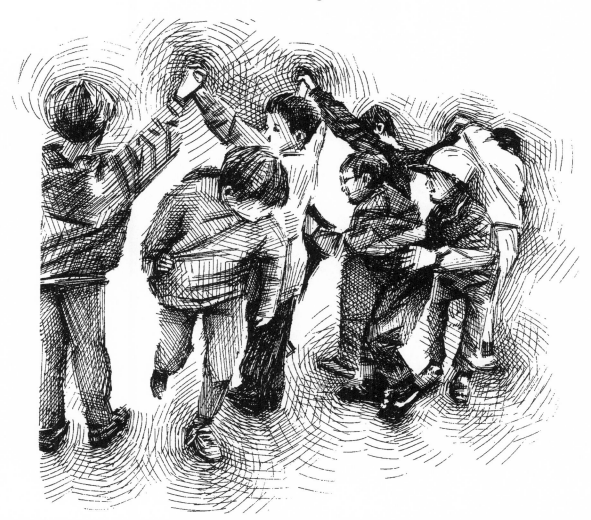

All the children hold hands up high in a circle so that one child can weave in and out, moving under the upraised arms. At the appropriate time in the song, she will stand behind a child, tapping her on the shoulder. This child is now first and the other child will hold on to her waist as they keep the song going in and out of the upraised arms of the circle.

Awareness

Five children will wait while the rest of the class holds hands in a circle. The task is for the five children to try to get into the circle while the children in the circle try to keep them out.

Children trying to get in, look for ways to do this. Children holding hands, be gentle as you try to keep them out.

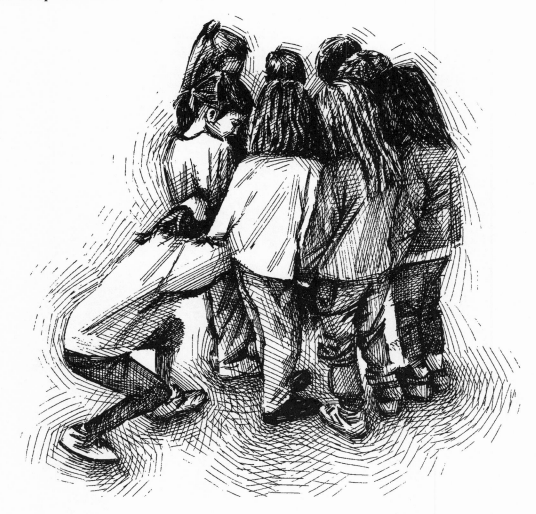

Discussion

How did it feel to try to get in while you were kept out? Did you try very hard to get in? Did you look for all possible openings? Did you band together as a group to try and break in? Did you give up at one point?

If they succeeded in getting into the circle: How did it feel to get into the circle when the group was trying to keep you out?

Try this same exercise with the five children in the middle of the circle trying to get out. Do all you can to keep them in without being rough.

What can you do with these opposites? I will leave some space for you to jot down some ideas.

You may think of using individual parts and then the whole body in dance to express these concepts. Partners and whole groups may be appropriate for some concepts. Possibly, some props will extend your lesson or in some cases things in the room can be used.

Smooth and Jerky

    Stop and Go

Exciting and Calming

    Forward and Backward

Cold and Hot

    Hard and Soft

Long and Short

    Straight and Round

Loud and Soft

    Rough and Smooth

First and Last

    Right and Left

CATCHING AND LETTING GO

Fingertips

Face your partner and touch fingertips only.
Close your eyes and let your fingertips dance together.
Let the rest of your body move as much as possible while fingertips touch, keeping your feet in place.
Let's see the many ways you can dance with your partner.

Now, very gently, let go.
Keep your arms, hands, fingers and body dancing.
Remember to keep your eyes closed.
Think to yourself about how you feel without your partner.
We will verbally share our feelings later.
Still dancing with your eyes closed, try to find your partner's fingertips once more and continue your dance.

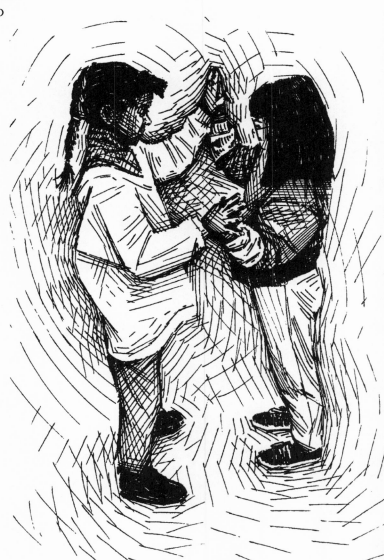

How do you feel now that you have found each other again?

Continue your dance.

Let go of your partner's fingertips again while you keep your arms dancing.

Find each other again.

Now open your eyes while continuing your dance.
Let go and dance around the room.

Make believe that you are trying to catch a star.
Go ahead and catch one.

Let it go.
Catch a soft cloud.

Let this go.
Keep your dance going while you are catching and letting go.

Catch a rainbow.
Let it go.

Catch a bunch of flowers.
Let them go.

Add your own things to catch and let go.

Catch a friend gently.
    And let go.
        Catch another friend.
            And let go.
                Catch another friend.
                    And let go.

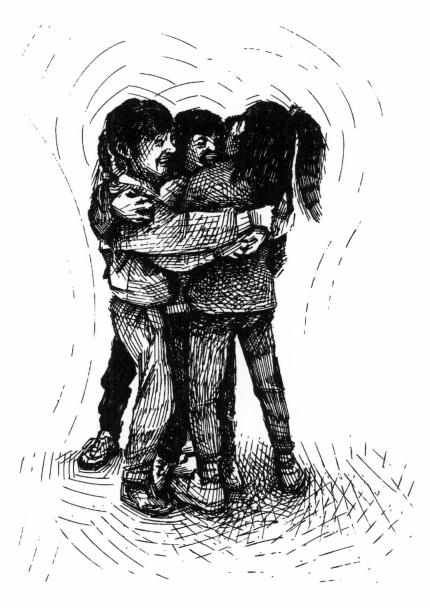

Discussion

How did it feel when you let go of your partner's fingertips?

    How did it feel when you found each other again?

        How did it feel when we were catching and letting go of things and each other?

        Which felt better to you, catching or letting go? Why?

OPEN–CLOSED

For Children with Special Needs

The following is an open-closed movement experience that was used with a group of three- to five-year-olds with an array of serious disabilities. The opening and closing of the body is how we sign for open and closed. Therefore, working with open and closed movements leads naturally to learning sign language. It became an easy and integrated way to use total communication to teach nonverbal children the language for spatial concepts by connecting the action to the word while learning to sign it.

> Let's open our hands—now close.
>
> O p e n , close, o p e n , close.
>
> Clenching and unclenching our fists,
>
> Clasping and unclasping our fingers.
>
> Flinging open our arms and then hugging our bodies.
>
> O p e n , closed, o p e n , closed.
>
> How about our legs?
>
> O p e n , closed, o p e n , closed.
>
> Our mouth.
>
> Our whole body.

Mark, a child with attention deficit hyperactivity disorder (ADHD), was not interested. He threw his body flat on the floor with arms flung open. I saw this as an opportunity to turn this acting-out behavior into a purposeful activity. I took Mark's hands.

> *Good, Mark. You are open.*
> **Then I pulled his arms to his chest, closing his body.**
> *Now you are closed.*
> **Mark threw his body back.**
> *Good, Mark, that is open!*
> *Now closed.*

Once again I pulled him closed. As Mark became aware of the game and that he was doing a "good job," he began to be less resistant to the activity.

Another child who is profoundly developmentally delayed and has restricted movement spontaneously moved his legs and arms open and closed after an adult modeled the motion and manipulated his body. Often the happy involvement of the group encourages a child who ordinarily finds it too difficult to participate.

A group of six children with autism and five adults held hands to form a circle. To show open and closed, we first made a large circle. Then we took little running steps toward the center to become closed.

Now we are closed.

We stayed there for a few movements so that the children could feel the contact and closeness of others.

Okay, let's become open and large again. Open up!

Looking around at the children I sensed that they were more aware of the group.

Let's close up again.

The children enjoyed this and cooperated in becoming both closed and close. The classroom teacher said that this was the first time these children showed awareness of others in the room.

Five-year-old Susie, who has Down's syndrome, spontaneously gave both of her hands to another child when I said "open."

That's a good idea. Let's work with partners.

O p e n ,

closed.

The partners hugged when I said "closed."

Using the children's ideas validates them and expands the lesson. I learn a great deal from the children; some of my best ideas are initiated by them.

John, who is neurologically impaired, resisted becoming the partner of another child, but he enjoyed working with an adult. He seemed to enjoy the social interaction and enclosure brought about by hugging. After a while, he became receptive to doing the same thing with a peer. Most children can perform this activity, regardless of ability.

Props

We sometimes use props to expand the lesson. For many children who have no socialization skills, props are a way of connecting them to others. They accept being next to each other in a common activity with a common goal.

Ropes

We placed a rope around the outside of our circle and held onto it from behind, saying "open." Then, crowding into the middle of the circle, we said "closed." The rope helped the children see open and closed shapes more objectively.

Later that day, four-year-old Mark, who is nonverbal and classified with ADHD, brought me the rope. I placed the rope around the two of us and played open and closed. He was all smiles. Mark had been in school for six months and this was the first time he had asked appropriately for an activity.

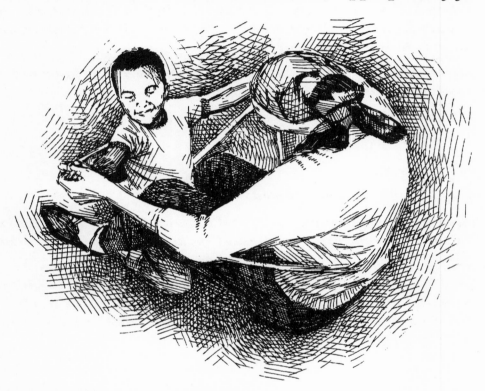

I have found that the more that children believe they are good people, the more pride they take in their accomplishments and the more they begin to establish positive and appropriate communication with others.

What can a rope become?

Your rope can become anything.
> It can be a line.
>> Make a line with your rope.
>>> Your line can be straight or round.
>>>> It can be held up in the air or down on the floor.
>>>>> Partners can make a straight line with a rope, each holding one end.

Twist your rope to make shapes that you know, such as a triangle, or letters, such as *V* or *W*. If you step on the middle of the rope and hold each end up high with your hands, you are making the letter V.

Parachute

Everyone may stand on the parachute. Now we are going to put the edges of the parachute over you so that you can be closed and immediately open it so that you can be open.

Closed, o p e n , closed, o p e n .

It's like playing peek-a-boo.

If someone doesn't like the idea of being closed up, even for a split second, that child shouldn't have to be involved.

We are in a constant search for modes of processing that will integrate concepts for the children. When one avenue is blocked we simply continue until we contact other receptive senses. Our involvement with props helps expand the multisensory approach by incorporating additional tactile and visual experiences.

Hoops

Allow for free exploration of the hoops for as long as there is interest.

Hop into and jump out of the hoops.
  Stand on them.
    Walk around the hoops.
      Put your arm through.
        Place the hoop behind you, in front of you, next to you.

Stand in the middle of your hoop.
  Put it above you and then below your knees.
    Go into the red, blue, yellow, purple, orange and green hoops.
      How many people in each hoop?

Create a dance with your hoop.
  What else can you do with your hoop?

Objects

Open and close all possible things in the room such as the doors, drawers and different objects.

Opening

I continued with a relaxation experience "opening." It is a gentle reinforcement for closed and open. Each teacher closed a child up tight with arms wrapped around them for a few seconds. We said "all closed up." As slowly as possible we opened each child. We lifted their heads, opened their legs and arms and laid them down, stretching them out. The children enjoyed this soft unfolding. They allowed themselves to be opened and manipulated. They lay on the floor content and relaxed. We had quiet music playing to set the emotional tone. We then placed the children in pairs where they gently experienced this unfolding with each other in a cooperative way.

Many activities that begin with teacher and student as partners can also lead to child-child partners and then to total group interaction. Children learn a good deal from each other and have the opportunity to initiate their original ideas. Children find each other stimulating and their joint activities give them opportunities to be spontaneous.

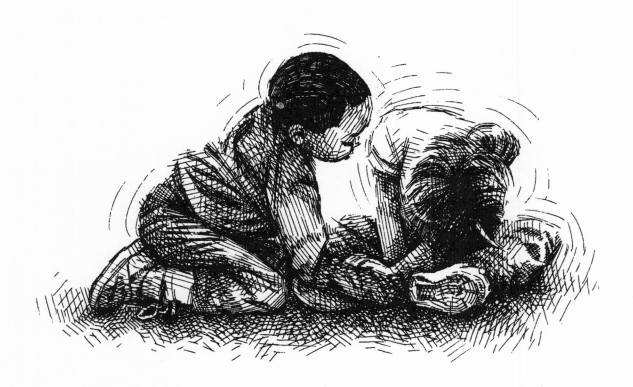

One child unfolded his partner who was severely developmentally delayed and had no language or eye contact. She allowed her partner, however, to manipulate her into an open position, a positive experience for both children. The opening experience created new ways for the children to touch and be touched and become more aware of each other.

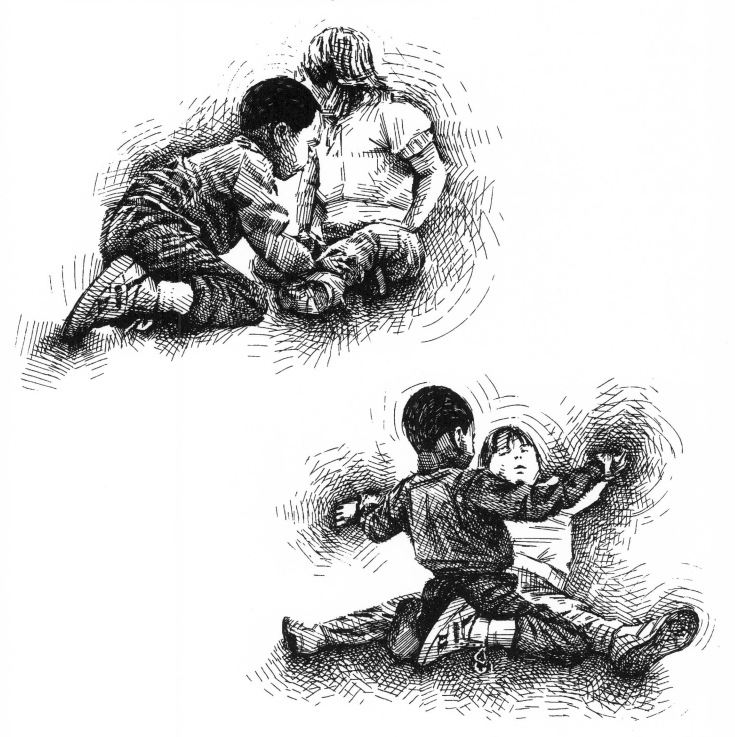

ACKNOWLEDGING

Feelings
Body Image
Self-Image
Others
Environment

Responding
 Reacting
  Joining
   Applauding
    Appreciating
     Thanking
      Recognizing
       Praising
        Understanding
         Supporting
          Accepting

Approving
 Celebrating
  Respecting
   Cherishing
    Admiring
     Treasuring
      Crediting
       Honoring
        Praising
         Touching
          Sensing
           Connecting

Showing Empathy, Kindness, Sympathy and Tenderness

EXPRESSING FEELINGS

Say, "No, I don't want to!" with different feelings, such as:

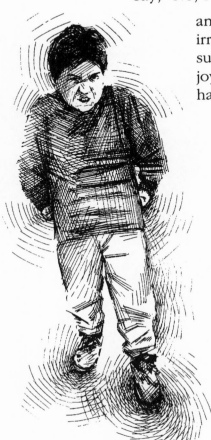

anger	boredom	excitement
irritation	grief	loneliness
surprise	sleepinesss	silliness
joy	fright	shyness
happiness	sad	
	disappointment	
	embarrassment	
	grumpiness	
	nervousness	
	depression	
	hurt	
	calm	
	exhaustion	
	relief	

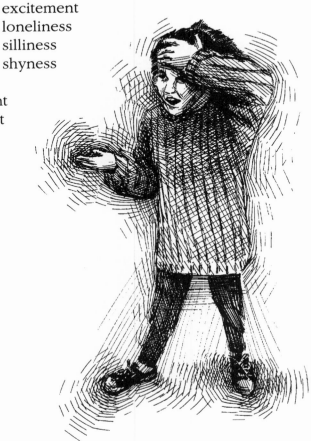

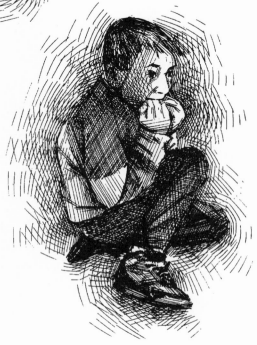

Now let's express these feelings nonverbally using our whole bodies. Some of us can watch our friends expressing these feelings with their bodies and guess which feeling they are revealing.

Try expressing these feelings with a partner.

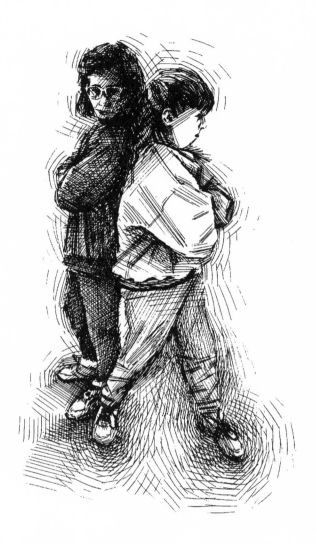

Discussion

How did it feel to be able to say, "I don't want to!"

Do you remember any time you wanted to say, "I don't want to" and didn't think you could say it?"

Do you remember any time you did say, "I don't want to" and then you were sorry you said it?

Are there any other feelings you would like to explore by yourself or with a partner?

Stories

Act out a story you know well in a different way, such as "Little Red Riding Hood" or the "Three Little Pigs" from the point of view of the wolf or "Hansel and Gretel" from the point of view of the stepmother or the wicked witch.

What are you feeling as this character?

Photographs

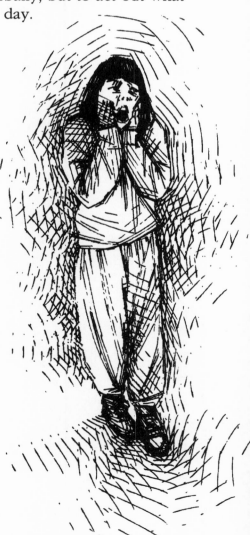

Bring in an old or recent photograph from your family album. We will spread them out and walk around, looking at them all.

Now come back to your own photograph. Those who would like may take turns telling a story about what may have been happening that day or something about yourself at the time the photograph was taken. Don't forget to include what you may have been feeling in the photograph.

You may choose not to share verbally, but to act out what might have been happening that day.

For Older Children

Sit in groups of three to share your photograph stories.

Goals

Choose two goals in the room that are far apart from each other. It may be the door, window, or desk. Anything you wish. Go toward that goal with the different feelings I will be calling out.

Go with determination.
Go with hesitation.
Go with grief or sadness.
Go with joy or happiness.
Go with fear.
Go with bravery.
Go with great energy.
Go with tiredness.

What other feelings can you use
to go toward your different goals?

CLAY AND PLAY

Warm Up

Let's warm up our bodies. Move your head in as many different ways as you can. Now your shoulders, arms and fingers. Great! Now include your back and waist. How about your feet, knees and legs? Begin to move throughout the room to the music any way you like. Bend, twist and stretch your body in all directions. Good!

Now let's come over to all these materials and choose many different colors of clay, feathers, sticks, construction paper and markers. We will just play and experiment with these materials, forming the clay into different shapes. It doesn't have to look like anything you know, but eventually it may begin to remind you of different things, such as an imaginary playground. Place your images on a large sheet of construction paper, choosing your own color. When you are all finished, we will walk around the room and look at all the colorful images you have made.

Stories

Now go back to your clay sculpture and create a fanciful story about it. The rest of the class will listen. When you are finished with your story you may ask the class if they have any ideas about what your sculpture reminds them of and let them add to your story.

We can divide into groups of four to do this so that many of you will have a chance to tell your story.

After we tell the stories, I would like to bring all the colored construction paper together so that we can see all the shapes as if it were one big story.

How about someone making up a story about what we see as a class clay sculpture? A few of you can do this and we can all add onto the story as it is being told.

Passive Active

Using the passive active game from *A Moving Experience,* a few of you can sculpt the rest of the class into the story that was just told or spontaneously move into a story sculpture as the story is told.

SCARVES

Scarves are a versatile prop. We can reinforce the names of body parts by throwing scarves in the air and catching them on different body parts. We can use them to learn about and feel colors. We can dress up and create spontaneous stories. Scarves always seem to inspire joyful, colorful and creative happenings that can be repeated.

Under the Scarves

One day the children decided to bury each other. One child lay down in the middle of many fallen scarves and placed them on himself. Spontaneously the other children began to throw more scarves on him until he was completely covered. We then began to give positive affirmations about the child who was buried.

Isn't he handsome?
    I like Craig.
        I like to play with Craig.
            He is so creative.
Walk around Craig, saying what you like about him.

Ask Craig which color he wants on his face.
    Red? Okay. Here is a nice, bright red.
Gently let the scarf float onto
    Craig's face.
Now that you are buried you
    can slowly stand up and let
the scarves fall away from you.
    Who else wants a turn to
get buried?

Standing

Maybe you prefer to stand while the others drape the scarves on and around you. Positive affirmations can still be made.

The facilitator can model this gently and slowly so that it becomes a very peaceful, loving game. Usually all of the children want a turn at this.

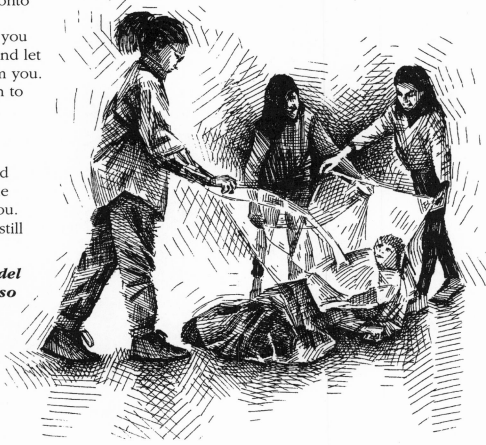

Your Favorite Color

Choose your favorite color for this moment. Dress up in lots of scarves and fabrics using only that color.

How would you describe your color? Use as many words as you can think of to describe that color. For example, red may feel like hot and lots of energy. Begin to let those feelings into your body and move throughout the space feeling your color.

You may want to team up with a partner and share your feelings and fantasies about your color. You can create a fantasy story about your color to share with your partner.

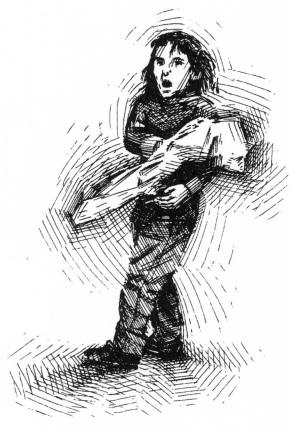

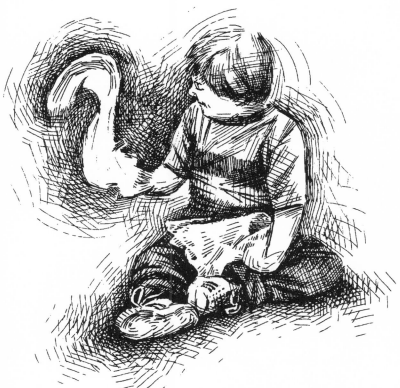

For Children with Special Needs

A few children with whom I have worked had little or no verbal language. They usually self–stimulated by making patterns in the air with their hands. However, placing scarves around their wrists turned the hand patterns into dancing scarves. Watching the scarves move seemed to stimulate them into moving more purposefully.

MY HERO

Imagery

Get yourself into a comfortable position and close your eyes. Think of someone you admire, someone for whom you have a lot of respect. Create a picture of this person in your mind. Imagine this person doing something very brave, such as helping someone in trouble or performing a remarkable feat. Maybe this person is able to overcome great personal obstacles.

There are many different kinds of heros. Make a movie of your hero in your imagination. Notice where your hero is and what he is doing or wearing. Are you with your hero? Think of something you and your hero can do that is the same.

Ask your hero to come and stay with you.
How do you look when you do something wonderful?

Imagine yourself as the hero.

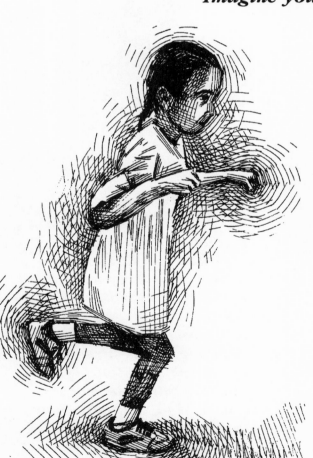

What do *you* do that is great?
Where are you when you perform this heroic act?
Are there other people there?
Look around you and notice where you are. Feel how proud you are!
Make a movie of yourself doing brave and wonderful deeds.
Notice other people who are with you and how proud they are of you.
Take a few moments to enjoy your glory.

Now I will count to three to bring you back and please bring your hero with you.

One: Be aware of where you are in this room and who else is in the room with you. Be aware of the floor or chair you are lying or sitting on.

Two: Begin to stretch your hands and arms, neck and shoulders and legs.

Three: Begin to open your eyes in your own time and get accustomed to the light and the room again.

Your hero is still with you. *You* are the hero: Tell me some words that describe how you feel as a hero.

Some answers were

brave	*happy*	*smart*
athletic	*powerful*	*awesome*
sweating	*strong*	*laughing*
beautiful	*rich*	*afraid*
talented	*friendly*	*artistic*
nice	*funny*	*famous*
loving	*scared*	

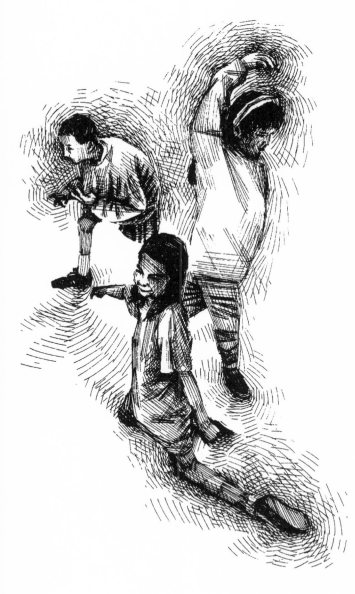

Movement

Stand up and move around the room feeling these words as I say them. You are the hero. Feel these words in your whole body and let those feelings move you around the room.

Now I will be quiet and let you say the words that come into your mind as you meet each other in the room.

Feel the words you say and express them in your body.

Now freeze.

Say, "I am my own hero. I am brave."

Continue dancing through the room as your brave hero and freeze.

Say, "I am my own hero. I am intelligent." Continue dancing through the room as your intelligent hero and freeze.

Say, "I am my own hero. I am strong."

Continue dancing through the room as your strong hero and freeze.

Say, "I am my own hero.

I am beautiful.

I am handsome."

Discussion

Let's sit down together and find out who are some of your heroes.

dancer	*Batman*
policeman	*Olympic figure skater*
Spider woman	*runner*
Superwoman	

The Hero was created by Nancy Crafts for her final project in the author's course, Therapeutic Applications of Dance Therapy in Education at Hahnemann University.

BOUNCING NAMES

This is a good way for children to learn one another's names. The children stand or sit in a circle. One person has a large bouncing ball. Usually the children know at least one other person's name.

Bounce the ball to someone in our circle and say her name. That person will then bounce it to someone else and say his name. We will do this until we think we know everyone's name.

Variations

Speed up the process as we begin to learn one another's names.

Perhaps you may be able to throw the ball instead of bouncing it.
Or sit down and roll it.

After you know each other's names, pass the ball quickly to the person on your left, saying her name. Let the ball pass all around the circle. Then do the same passing the ball to the right.

Find other ways to pass the ball. How about passing it behind your back or bounce it under your leg to the next person?

How about pushing the ball with your foot and catching it with your foot?

We will add a second ball and then a third so that several of you will get your name called at the same time.

Say your own name, bouncing the ball to each syllable. Say your name and how you are feeling as you bounce the ball.

Stand in the middle of the circle and call someone's name as you throw the ball in the air. That person must catch it before it bounces. You can make it a little easier by allowing one bounce.

Make two facing lines. Bounce the ball back and forth down the aisle.

Can you think of another way to use the ball while we learn each other's names?

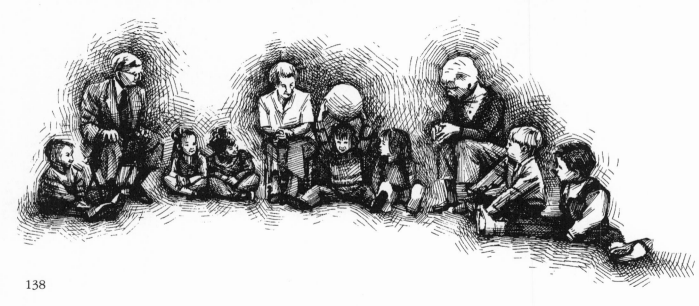

For Children with Special Needs

While in a circle, pass a ball to the next child rhythmically while saying that child's name. If a child is unable to pass the ball, the teacher can place it in her hands and then move it on to the next child.

In one class of special children, a child reached for the ball for the first time indicating the beginning of communication and focus.

Being present in the group can enhance socialization skills even if motor and mental skills are limited.

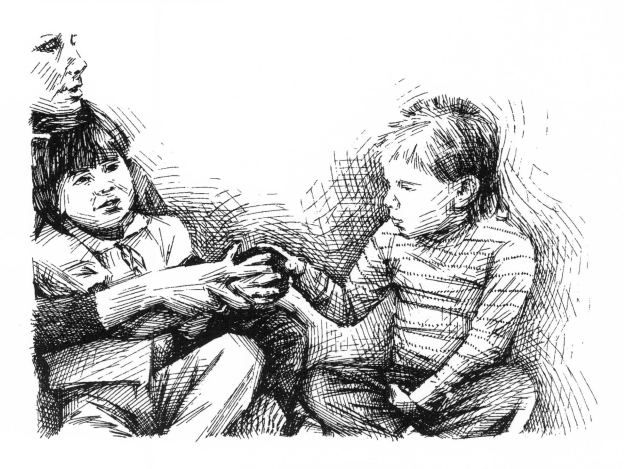

Variations

Hold the ball. Put it up in the air.
Now down in your lap.
Up in the air.
Down in your lap.
Say "up" and "down" as we put the ball up and then down.
Very good!

NAMES AND FEELINGS

I Feel, She Feels, He Feels

I'm Lawrence and I feel _____.
   Create a movement to show how you feel.
Everyone else will say, He's Lawrence and he feels _____.
   You copy his movement. *Next!*
I'm Robert and I feel _____. He's Robert and he feels
_____. Go around in a circle until everyone has had a turn.
   Keep going around to see how your feelings change.
Let's go faster this time.

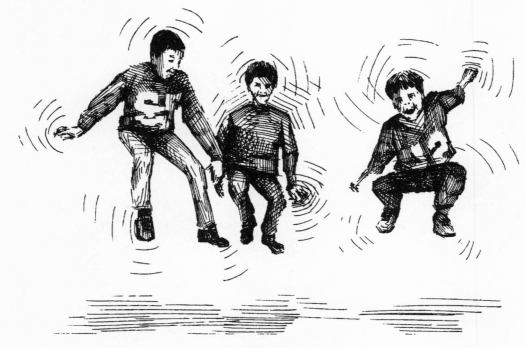

Variation

   Create a movement that will say how you feel without speaking and pass that movement around the circle as quickly as possible.
   One person begins and then turns to the next person to share his gesture with her. The person that just received the gesture can change it slightly and give it to the next
   person and so on until it comes back to the original person.
You can go around doing this as many times as attention span will allow.

Sound Variation

   Create a sound that everyone will repeat that expresses how you feel. Let everyone in the circle have a turn, as in I feel, he feels.
   This experience evolved during one of Sandra Mussey's workshops on developing intuition.

Pictures

Spread pictures that express different feelings on the floor. Let children choose pictures of how they are feeling.

140

MAGICIAN

I am a magician.
I am turning you into a
                    snake.
                        tiger.
                            monster.

You are _____.
                color

Be aware of how you are
feeling.

You are _____.
                feeling

Ask yourself why and
how you are feeling
that way.

LEARNING ABOUT ME

Art

Place a photograph of yourself in the middle of a paper. Now cut out pictures from magazines that describe you. You may also draw things that you relate to. Write under the pictures what you are doing. For example you may write, "I am being a good friend," or, "I like to play the piano," or, "I like soccer."

Writing and Movement

Write a paragraph about yourself. You may use the ideas from the pictures you just cut out from the magazine that describe you.

    You may write about what you are good at

        or what you like to daydream about

            or what you want to be when you grow up

                or what you like to do when you relax

                    or what you like to do in the

                                    summer,

                                        winter,

                                          spring

                                              or fall.

Now get a partner. Take turns acting out what you wrote. Can your partner guess what you said?

Now your partner will create her own movement and act out something she especially likes about you. Guess what was acted out. Take turns doing this and then share your feelings about this activity.

Group Sharing

Place these collages and paragraphs around the room. Those who would like to may read their stories to the class.

Write Your Own Book

What stories can you show about your day?
    We will guess what you are doing.
        This is me going on my bike to the game. Then this is me saying hi to my friend
            and this is me playing soccer and this is me who won the game.

For young children, the teacher can write it as it is told. The children may also find
pictures in magazines that illustrate what they want to write about and paste the pictures
in their books.

Have someone else sculpt your story using as many of your classmates as they need
while you read it.

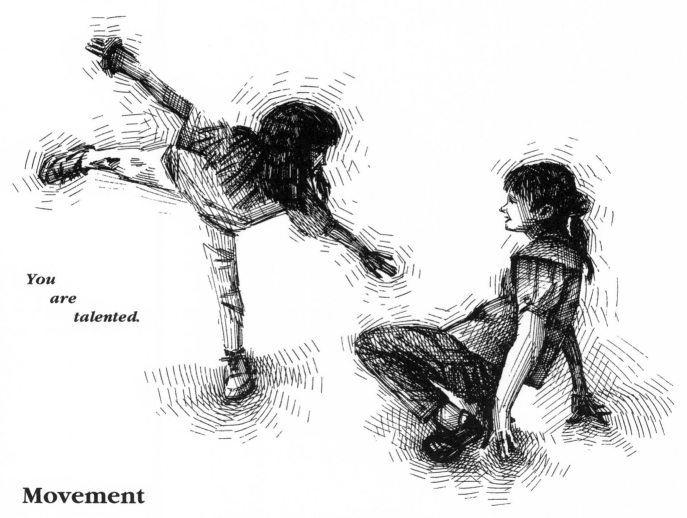

You
    are
        talented.

Movement

They could also write the "Me Book" or "How I Spend My Day Book."
    This book can then be experienced in movement as someone else reads it aloud.
        Or the author can read and have the class act it out.

Thank you Leigh Gellman

SELF-AWARENESS
OTHER AWARENESS

Body Awareness

Walk around the room, listening to your body. Be aware of any feelings or twitches.
   Be aware of where your shoulders are.
Are your shoulders pushed backward or forward?
   Is one shoulder lower than the other?
In what direction are your feet pointed?
   Do they point inward or outward? Are you walking on the balls of your feet or on the heels?
   Choose one of these parts of your body that you are aware of and exaggerate what you are doing.
   Now bring it back the way it was.
Exaggerate it again.
   For example, if your shoulders are slightly forward, exaggerate so that they are extremely pushed forward.
   Be aware of how it feels when you exaggerate the position of that part of your body. Does it feel different when you go back to your normal position?

Exaggerating Your Walk

Do your worst walk possible.
   Maybe a part of your body is
      sticking out in an
         exaggerated way.
Maybe your feet are very turned in
   or your knees are touching
      or your arms are swinging
         out of control.
Can you think of anything?

Now walk normally, being aware of whether you are exaggerating your movements even a little bit.

You may want to consciously straighten your toes to face forward or straighten your back or anything else, to improve your posture.

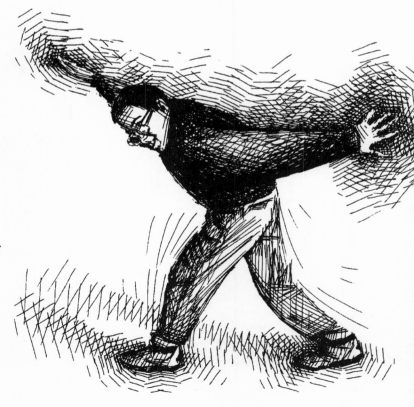

Group

Form two lines and then sit down. Everyone is sitting across from someone else, leaving a space large enough for someone to walk through.

Each person can have a turn to walk down the aisle and the rest of you will describe what you notice about that person. Call out what you notice. Try not to be judgmental. Observers may look for the following:

Listen to the sounds of her feet. How quickly or slowly is she walking?
　Are her toes pointed outward, inward or straight ahead?
　　Does she seem to hold back or is she going forward?
　　　Does she move as if she is light and airy or strong and into the ground?
　　　What else can you see about how she walks?
Is she taking her time or does she seem in a hurry?
　How long are her steps?
　　Does she take short, quick steps or long, slow steps?
　　　Do her arms swing freely or do they stay somewhat still?
　　　How far do the arms swing, going back and forth?
Does she pick up or slide her feet?
　Does she seem to walk more on the balls of her feet or more on her heels?
　　Is the walk smooth or irregular?
　　　What parts of the body seem stiff and which parts seem loose?
　　　What else do you notice?

This is a difficult task for the walker because people are watching you and describing the way you walk. You may feel self-conscious so try to walk as naturally as you can. Your walk is not wrong or right, it is simply your individual walk and we are learning to observe.

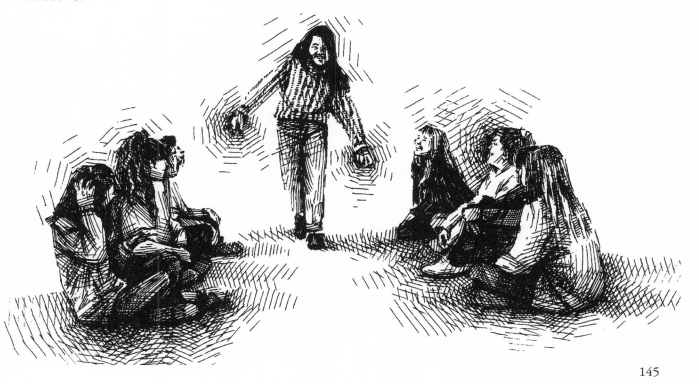

Partners

Choose a partner. Follow her or him around the room.

Try to imitate your partner's walk. Be aware of the things we talked about in group as you try to walk the same way as your partner does.

Do this for a while or until you have successfully copied your partner's walk.

I experienced partners in Sandra Mussey's intuition workshop.

Variation

As a variation, let your partner teach you his very own walk.

It helps to hold hands to get your partner's rhythm.

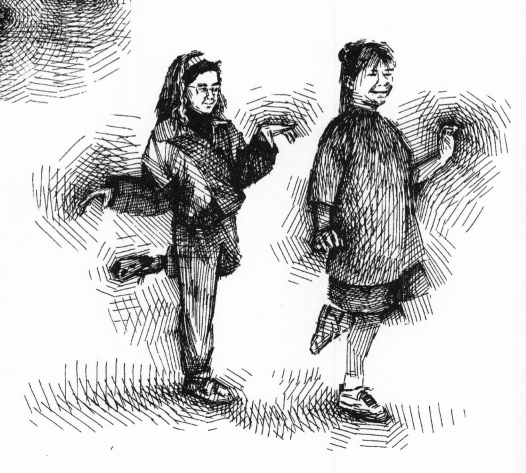

Face Your Partner

Stand on opposite sides of the room and face your partner. Those of you who followed will demonstrate your partner's walk. Partner number one, how does it feel to have someone walk the way you do? Do you recognize your walk? If not, how do you think your partner has to change to make the walk more like yours? Partner number two, do you agree?

Mirrors and Videotapes

Use mirrors or videotapes to let participants see their own ways of walking.

Imagination Walking

Imagine you are in a place of worship such as a church or synagogue. How will you walk?

Imagine you are in school. How will you walk?
Imagine you are on the playground. How will you walk?
Imagine you are
at a family dinner
at Grandmother's house
at the doctor's office
at a museum or theater
at the library
on public transportation
at a friend's house
at your own house
under a low ceiling

Homework Assignment

Observe some people you know walking in various places. Describe something about their walking that you can recognize at a distance.

Describe them by shape and size of their body and speed of movement.

Listen to the sounds of people's feet in a building or in your home. Can you tell something about them? Do you know who they are even when you can't see them?

BODY COLLAGE

Dressing Up and Tracing

Here are some scarves, hats and other fabrics.
Get dressed up any way you like.

While you are decorated with the scarves, I will put on some music so you can dance to whatever you are feeling. This may help you decide how you want to shape your body when it is traced on a paper.

Lie down on a sheet of paper, large enough for your entire body to stretch out. Ask your friend to trace you. You can be in any position, with your legs spread apart or together. Your arms could be above your head, out to the side, down next to you or with your hands on your hips. Whatever you like. Just remember that only the parts of you that touch the paper will be traced.

Quietly sit by yourself with a bunch of your favorite magazines. Cut out pictures that interest you. You don't have to know why you like them or why you are interested in them. Just cut them out.

Now find a good place for them inside the outline of your body. When you like where you have placed them, paste them all on the paper. You may want to use markers to expand, change or add to your pictures.

Using markers or paints, color in any empty spaces.

You may want to go over the outline to make it more visible.

It is very effective to have the finished body collages taped around the room. Both children and adults have commented on how their images make them feel: Now the room really belongs to them.

We will visit each collage as its owner tells us about it. When we get to yours you may talk about the pictures and why you picked them or you may choose to say nothing. The rest of the class will admire and acknowledge you.

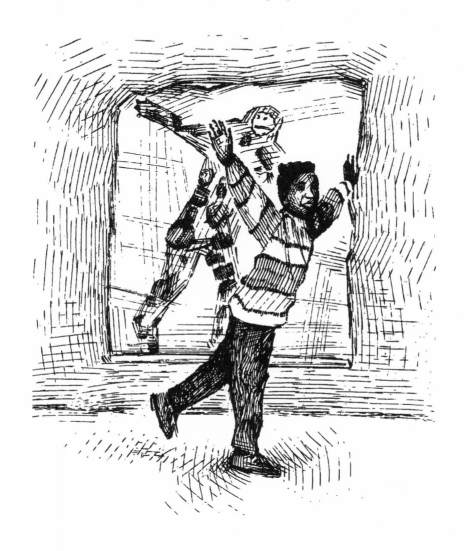

I Feel

Take turns choosing one picture on your collage. Shape your body into whatever you picked and say "I am a _____ and I feel _____."
The rest of the class will shape their bodies into the object and say, "Harlene is a _____ and she feels _____."

This experience developed out of a workshop with Sandra Mussey on intuition.

You can do this as long as time and attention span allow.

For Older Children

Now that your collage is finished, you may do some free writing outside your body out-line. Let the pictures of your collage stimulate you. You may write single words or short sentences. Be spontaneous; don't try to think of what to write. Let the words flow from you as if you were doodling.

For Younger Children

You can write for the children who are not able to do so, as they verbalize their feelings.

Young children find it easier and faster to use paint to fill in the spaces. This is a long process and is more successful if done over a period of time.

To save time, you can ask children to bring in pictures or even photographs from home.

Create a story from the pictures.

You can do this verbally in a spontaneous way. Children who are able may write their stories.

Dance your story as one child or the whole class reads what you wrote.

Develop a drama from your story, with you as the star. If you need others to help, the rest of the class can participate. You can also sculpt a group of children who will represent your story.

Positive Feedback

Have your body traced again, but this time let the whole group take turns placing the pictures and words that describe you. Group, please be positive, caring and supportive. *It is better to do this after the children have known each other for a while.*

Sharing

You may do this in pairs or as a whole group.

Read and talk about the pictures that were placed on your body collage.

Describe how it feels when others say what they think and feel about you.
    Do you agree?
        With which parts do you disagree?

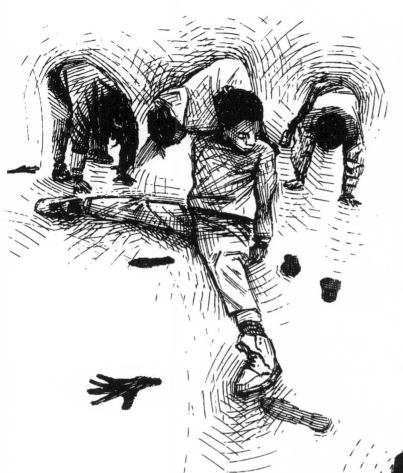

HANDS AND FEET

Trace your hands and feet. Cut the tracings out and place them all over the room.

Now move around, trying to put your hands and feet on the patterns.

Move every time the leader says, "Change."

Can you find a hand or foot that nobody else is on?

Are you getting all tangled up?

Try this with different colors. When I say "green," everyone has to find green hands and feet.

Great!

Now change to yellow.

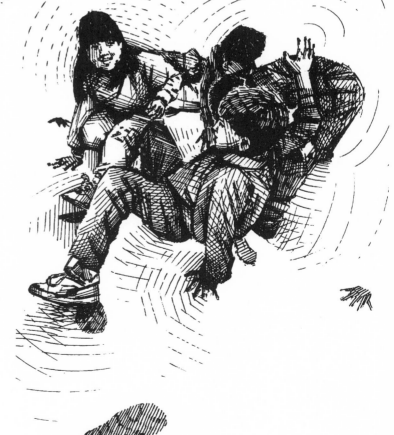

SHADOWS

Partners

One of you will be the sculpture and your partner will be your shadow. Shadow, lie down in front of your partner with your feet almost touching your partner's feet. Shape your body to reflect the exact position of your partner. Every time we say "Change," the sculpture will change shape and the shadow will try to follow.

Dance

In slow motion, the standing person will move his whole body while keeping feet planted in one spot. The shadow will follow. Standing partner, remember to move slowly so that your shadow can follow you.

Time of Day

Shadow, adjust your position in relation to your partner as I say what time it is and where the sun is in the sky.

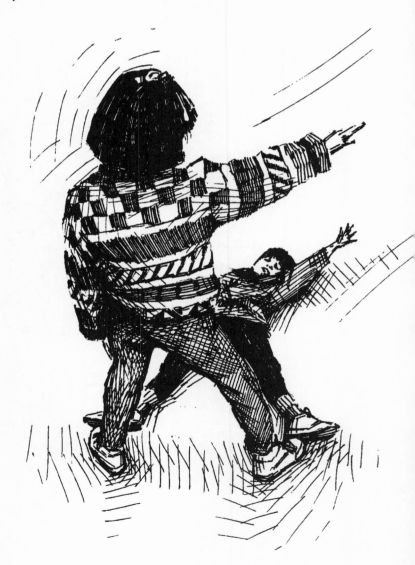

Art

Draw a picture of a person. Put black paper in back of it and cut out both papers. Place the black paper upside down, feet to feet, to create the picture of a person with his shadow.

GAMES

Games that are noncompetitive

can foster group awareness,

help generate leadership,

develop cooperation,

promote fun and enjoyment

and encourage bonding

among the players

GAMES

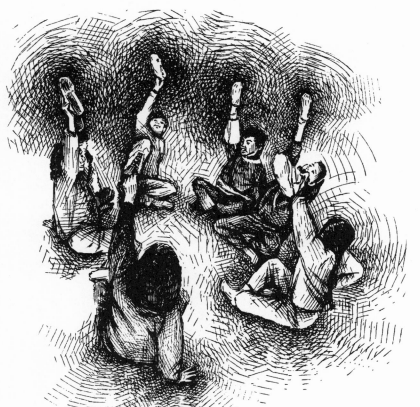

Pass the Shoe

This is my shoe.

Tell you what I'm going to do,
Pass it right on to you.

or

I will pass my shoe
   from me to you
      from me to you
         from me to you
I will pass my shoe
and this is what I'll do!

Everyone sit in a circle. Take off one of your shoes and hold it in your right hand.

As we say this rhyme, tap your shoe gently from right to left in front of you. When we say, "pass it on," you may pass it to the person next to you on the right (or left).

Continue this until your own shoe comes back to you.

Then hold up your shoe and say, "This is my shoe."

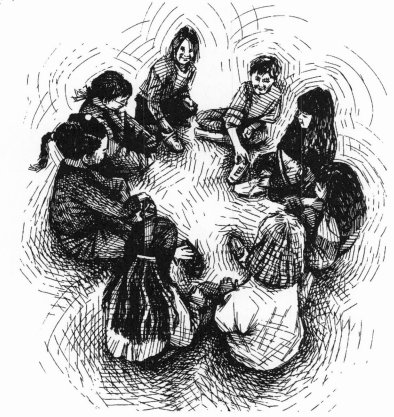

Car Wash

Everyone stand in a circle facing the same direction with legs spread apart. One person at a time crawls under the legs while being massaged on the back by each person she passes.

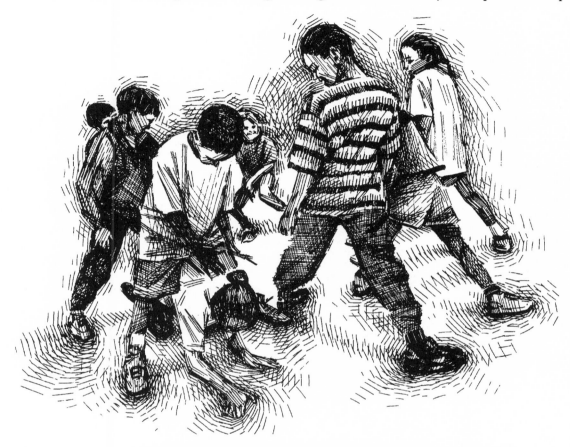

Commands and Obedience

Without talking, be the boss by using simple gestures. You may tell your followers to come, go, stop, sit, jump up, run, change direction, go over there, turn around or anything else you can think of without getting your followers hurt.

We will give as many of you a chance as there is time available. How does it feel to be a boss and have people do as you command? How does it feel to have to follow orders? When is it a good idea to follow orders and when is it not a good idea to follow orders?

Use Sound

Use your voice in a different way to direct movement. High pitched for moving up and low pitched for moving down. Sing loud for strong movements and then softly for gentle movements. Sing quickly for fast movement and slowly for slow movement.

Combine your hands and voice to create the movements you would like your group to perform.

Cradle Pass

As many people as needed, stand next to each other holding one player in a horizontal position.

With great care, pass that person down to the next standing person. The first person is now free to go to the end of the line and stand in place to hold the player.

This is a trust experience, so be very careful to hold your player gently and caringly.

You may add a smooth rocking motion as you hold and pass your friend.

The player may choose to close her eyes to really enjoy this holding by her friends.

You may use soft music to enhance this gentle cradle.

This would be safer to do on a mat.

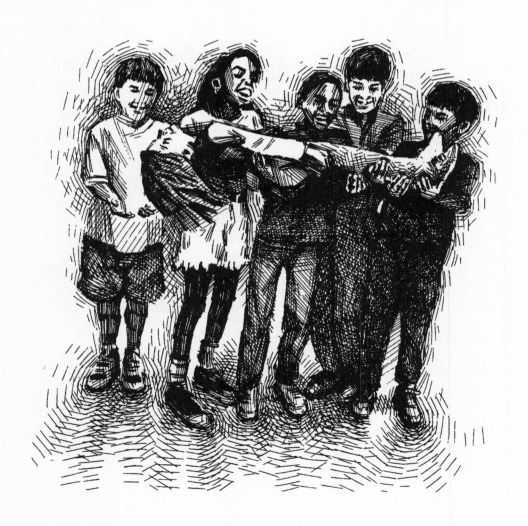

TRUSTING IMPROVISATION

Blind Walk

One person, the leader, will take her blindfolded partner around the room to explore and touch different objects and furniture. Try to figure out what the objects are as you investigate them. The purpose of this exercise is to expand sensory awareness as well as to be able to trust your partner. This is also an exercise in learning how to take care of someone. Leader, take good care of your partner and don't let anything hurtful happen to her or him. Give your blindfolded partner an opportunity to touch many different textures and shapes. Change roles so that each of you has the opportunity to be the one that is blindfolded as well as the leader.

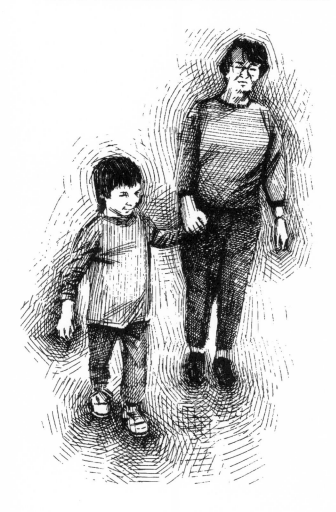
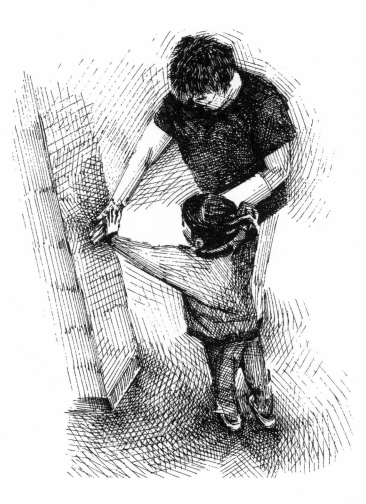

Circle of Friends

One person may go into the center of a small circle. We'll call you the dancer. Keep your feet together and fall forward, sideways and backward keeping your feet stationary. Your circle of friends will support and move you around. Let your body fall in any direction it is moved. You can try this with eyes open or closed. It is your choice.

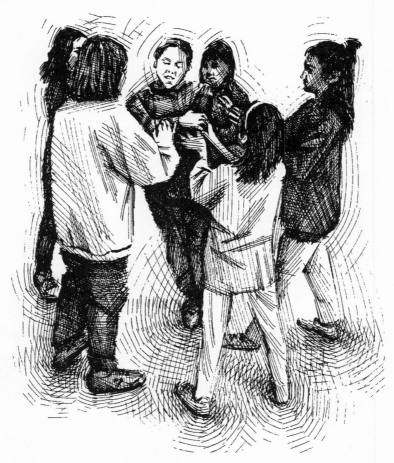

Improvisation

Let the circle open up so that the dancer can be moved around the room, allowing all present to help manipulate her. The dancer can be handed from person to person as she is moved about. Friends, be on the alert for where you have to be in the room to support the dancer.

Trio

Two of you may stand facing each other with room enough between you for a friend to stand facing either of you. The middle person will fall forward and backward for you to catch her and send in the opposite direction to your partner. Middle person make sure you keep your feet together in one place and see how much you can trust your partners. Partners, stay as close to the person in the middle as your comfort level allows. You may alter the space between you as you work.

Jelly Roll

About ten children may lie down shoulder-to-shoulder. The end child may roll over all the bodies until she comes to the end and lies down alongside the last child. The next person does the same until all have had a chance to do the jelly roll. At the start, leave enough room at the end for the children to continue adding on. This is a fun activity that makes the children laugh a lot. Make sure the bodies are very close together so that the child rolling doesn't fall between.

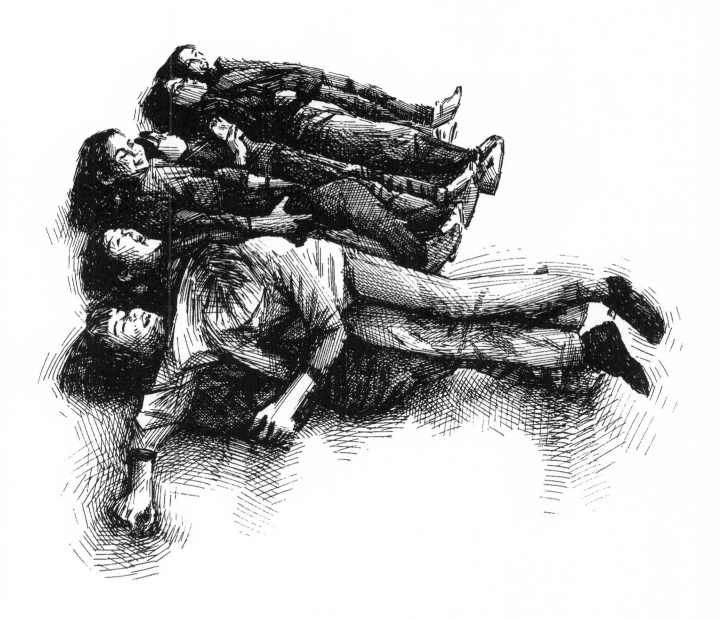

Rocking

One person may lie down on the floor. As many as can fit around that person may kneel down around her. Gently place your hands under the person and lift her. Slowly and gently rock her to and fro. The person experiencing this may close her eyes. While you are rocking your friend, you may say things about her you like. If she is feeling sick, such as complaining of a headache or a stomachache, you may say healing things, such as your stomach is feeling better or your head is now relaxed. Whatever you say, the intention is to make the person feel better.

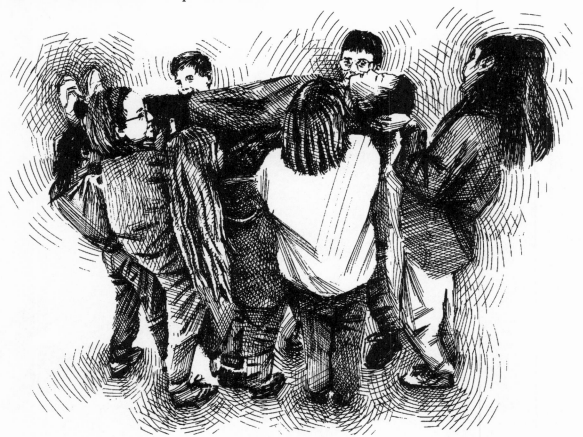

Tinickling

Here are two very long bamboo poles. One person on each end will take the poles in her hands. You will gently bang the poles on the floor and then together in rhythm. The dancer may stand between the poles, rhythmically jumping in and out without getting caught.

The pole holders can change the rhythms, banging the poles on the floor twice and together twice as in two by two or two by one. You can figure out different rhythms as your dancer gets used to jumping in and out.

Dancer, be creative in how you jump. You may want to turn in a circle as you jump. You may want to use your arms in a dance any way you can imagine.

Try crossing two pairs of poles and have the dancer move in and out of the square that is created by the crossing.

MORE CURRICULUM AREAS

Dance, poetry, art,

use of partners and group dances,

scarves and other props, performance, songs,

rhythm instruments, body sounds,

use of fast and slow, levels, range,

relaxation, fantasy, discussion, and images such

as animals can all be used in many of the curriculum areas.

Use these movement and arts possibilities to integrate

into your own lessons.

WIND AND LEAVES

Group

Let's sit in a circle, and one at a time, you may say as many words as possible to describe how a leaf may move.

Possibilities are

whirling, twirling, swirling, flying, floating, frisky, lingering, whipping, hurrying, rushing, whispering, settling, drifting, scurrying, scampering, gliding, drifting, shooting, bursting, lifting, rising, spinning, soaring.

I will write the words down for you to see.

Dance

Be a leaf responding to these words as I say them.
Use the entire space and your whole body as you dance these words.

Partners

One partner will be the wind and the other a leaf.
Wind, decide how strong or light you will be and tell your partner.
Leaf, respond by moving as the wind blows.

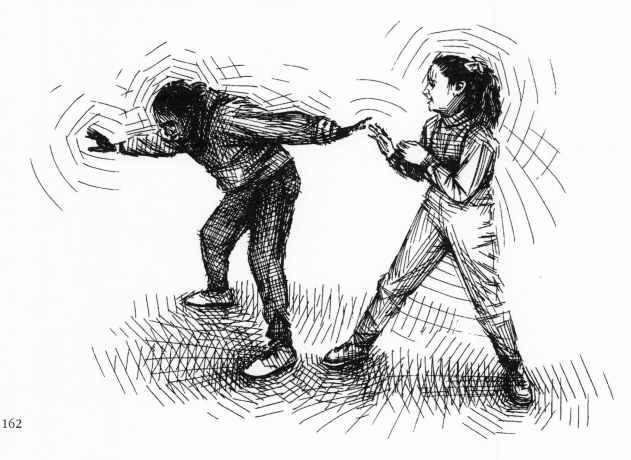

Poetry

Share words that describe the movement with your partner.

For example, if the wind is strong you may say that it is whirling, twirling and swirling. If the wind is gentle, you may say that the leaf is floating, flying and settling.

Create a simple poem together, using your descriptive words. Your poem can be as short as two lines or as long as eight.

One Child's Poem

The wind blew.
The leaf flew.
The wind blew strong.
The leaf whirled, twirled and swirled with all its might.
The wind was light.
The leaf rose, floated and settled without a fight.

Art

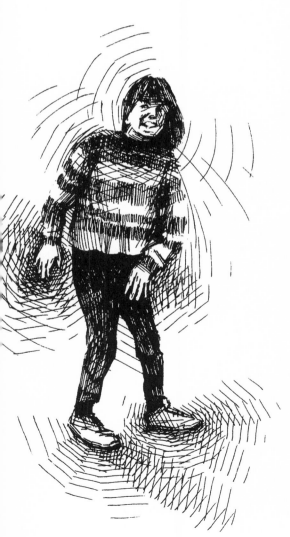

Have chalk of various colors and very large newsprint near by. Close your eyes and see yourself as the leaf moving through the room.

Now open your eyes and choose any colors you like. Let your arm move through the space as you envisioned in your mind's eye.

Now place your chalk on your paper and let your hand move in the same way. You are creating the leaf's movement.

Movement

Place these leaf papers all around the room.

Now find another partner. Take turns moving to each other's pictures. Each artist will observe his or her partner moving to the artist's picture.

Watch your partner's interpretation of your picture. Is the movement what you felt when you were making your picture?

Sharing

Sit down with your partner and talk about what you saw in each other's dances. Discuss what you saw and felt in your partner's art work and in your dance.

163

Scarves

Choose a few scarves of the same colors as your leaf picture. See the movements in your drawing and let the scarves re-create those movements in space. Practice the movements over and over until you can remember them.

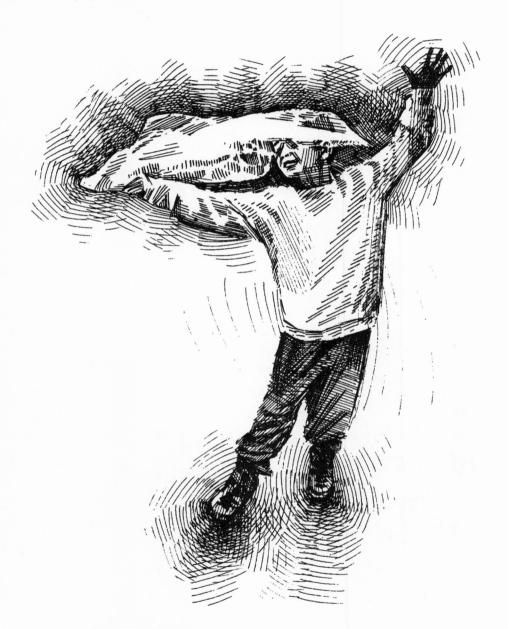

Performance

Five dancers at a time, take your places on the floor and begin your dance. Be aware of the others so that you don't bump into them.

They are beautiful dances. I can really see the wind affecting you.

164

CIRCLES

These circling activities were stimulated by my work with children with special needs and can also be used in the regular classroom.

Song
Tune from an old Irish folk song "Come Walking with Me."

> *Come circling with me*
> *Come circling with me*
> *Over the highway and down to the sea*
> *Come circling with me.*

The rhythm of this song brings everyone into the circling activities. Sing it over and over again, one activity flowing into another, always focused on circles.

> Make a circle in the air with your fingers.
> Now make a circle with your hand.

Mark, a child who is hyperactive, kicked his feet. I guided his foot to make circles in the air.

Mark, you are making a circle in the air with your foot.

> Let's each make a circle with our foot.
> Let's connect our circles to each other.
> Look! We are making one large

sculpture of connecting circles.
> "Come circling with me.
> Come circling with me."

Dance

How many ways can you move while your circles are connected to each other?

Make it a dance. Move up and down and around each other.

Find all the different ways you can create a circle dance.

Shape your body into gentle soft circles and feel roundness in your arms, back and legs.

We continue singing
> "Come circling with me."

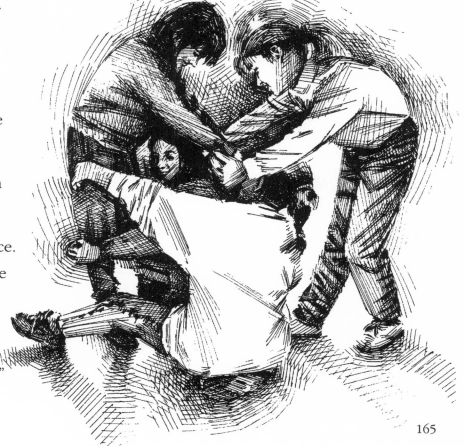

Props

Large Inner Tube

Let's sit on this large circle. Place a leg on either side.
Come bounce on the circle, come bounce on the circle.
What else can we do with this circle?
Put our feet into it. Good!
Two feet into the circle, two feet into the circle. Over the highway and down to the sea, two feet into the circle.
What else can we do with this circle?
Turn around in the circle, turn around in the circle.
Everyone out of the circle, everyone out of the circle.
Now let's bang on the circle with our fists.
One foot into the circle.
Now let's leave the circle.
I'll place this circle on end and we can all go through the circle.
Let's go through the circle, let's go through the circle.
Over the highway and down to the sea, let's go through the circle.
Everyone may go through, one at a time.

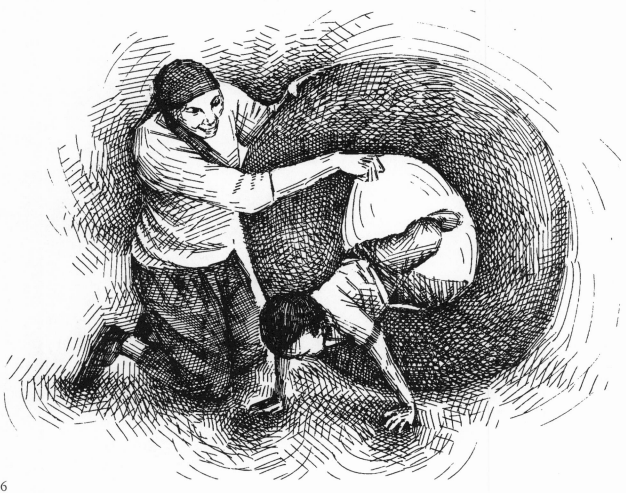

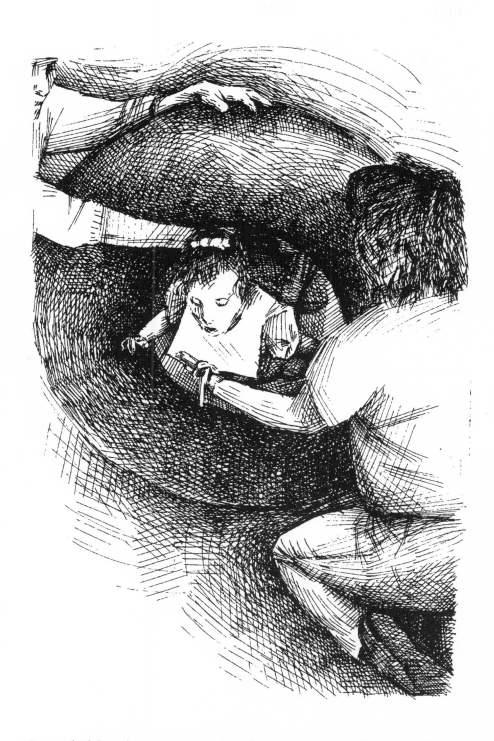

***One child, who was just beginning to be able to hold up her body, was passed
through the tire from one teacher to the next. The other children lined up for
their turns, over and over, as we continued our rhythmic song, never missing
a beat.***

Hoops

Everyone may get a hoop and sit inside the circle.
Let's move our hoops around our bodies as fast as we can. Now let's do that slowly.

Place your circle next to you, in back of you, in front of you, over your head, under your chin, up in the air, down near your knees.

Where else can we place our circle?

We can do anything with our circles. How about inviting a friend into your circle? Now we can sing "Two inside a circle, two inside a circle." We can do anything with our circle.

Let's go up and down inside our circle. Up and down in our circle, up and down in our circle. Hold hands with your partner and do a circle up-and-down dance.

Let's make our hoops go up and down.

How about making a hoop train? We can all hold onto the hoop in front of us with one hand while we hold onto our own hoop with the other hand and march around the room.

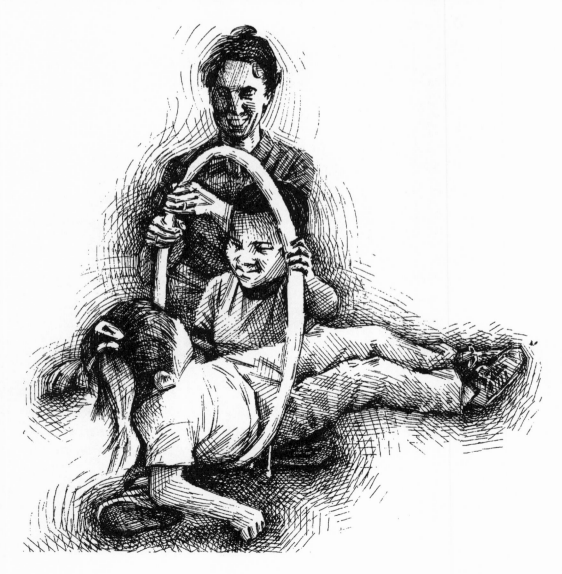

The hoops give the children a physical boundary and also help them to focus on circles.

What else can we do in our circles?

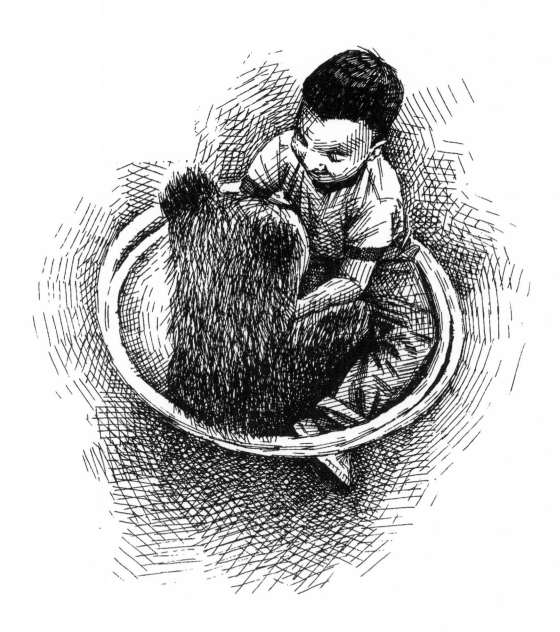

Scarves

Choose your favorite colored scarf and create circles in the air. Can you make little circles? How large can you make your circle with your scarf?

Ropes

Place a rope inside your circle in front of you and everyone may hold onto it. We can see and feel our circle.

With individual ropes for each person, we will shape our rope into a circle. Now we can dance in and out of our circle.

Sitting in a Circle

Teachers may sit behind the children to give added physical support and boundaries to those with special needs.

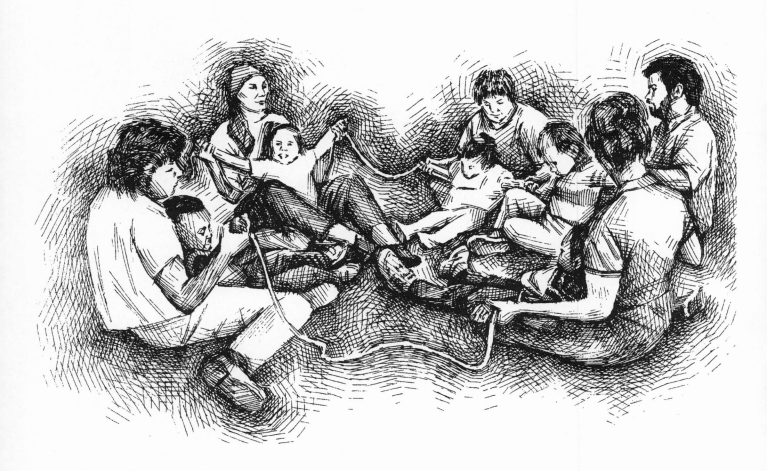

Elastic Ropes

Make a shape with your body using the rope. How about a triangle, a rectangle or a square? Can you make a different shape?

Let's make a group shape. The first person may begin and make a shape with your body and your rope. The next person can connect to some part of the first shape and make another form using the rope. Now someone else until we have a huge sculpture of different shapes.

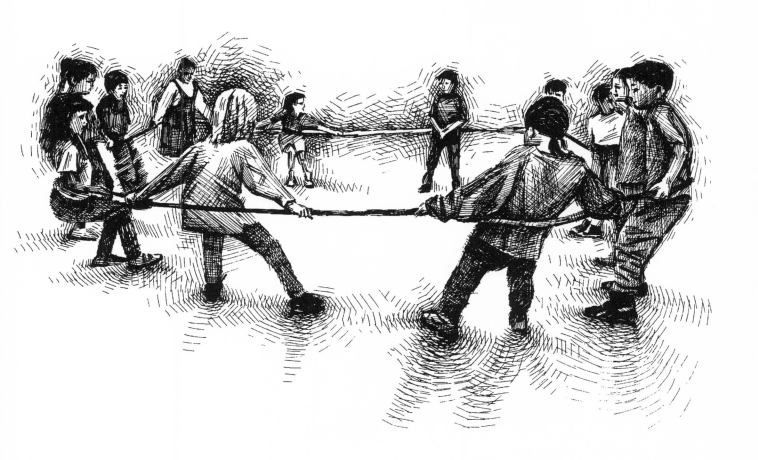

Co-Oper Band for a Trusting Circle

donated by Chime Time

Everyone may get inside this large stretch rope called the Co-Oper Band. Slowly we will allow our bodies to relax back on the rope while the rope holds us. We have to do this together as we are all balancing each other.

Crazy Shapes and Body Parts

Find another way to allow the rope to support you on different parts of your body. Be careful not to put the rope around your neck. Let's see all the different ways you can shape your body and all the places the rope can support you in our circle.

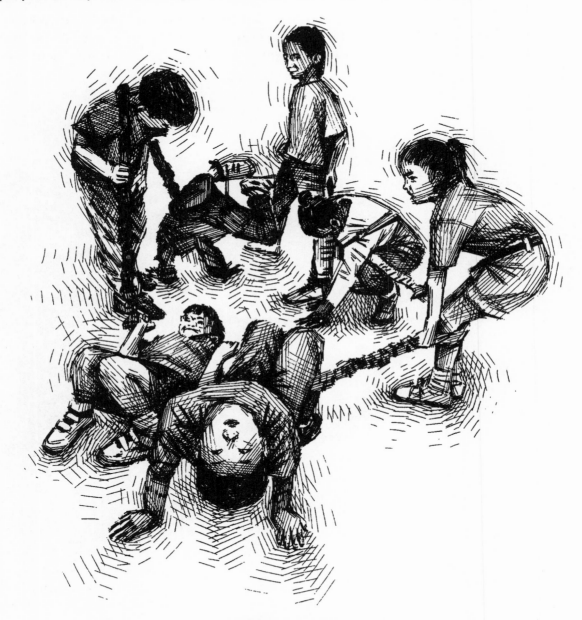

Shadow Play

We will set up a sheet in the middle of the room. You may go behind a few at a time. You'll have a light behind you to create circle shadows with your hoops. The rest of us will watch the circle show on the other side of the sheet. This is exciting, watching your show!!

In what other ways can you create circle shadows?

Relaxation

Teachers can partner with children who need special help.

We are going to find all of the circles on our bodies and trace them with our fingers.

Circles on our noses
Circles on our knees
Circles around our eyes
Circles on our cheeks
Circles on our chins
Circles on our ears
Circles on our elbows
Circles on our heels
Circles on our ankles
Circles on our stomachs
Circles on our shoulders
Circles on our heads

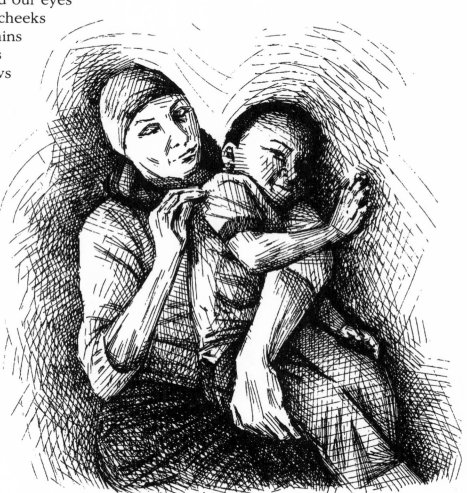

I have used the circle and the words for body parts over and over again, creating a hypnotic effect. In Mark's case, I traced circles on his body while he began to calm down.

Group Circle

Let's make a big circle. One at a time, children may come into the circle and do a circle dance. When you are finished, stand in front of another person in the circle to indicate it is his turn to go into the center. Continue until all who would like to have had a turn.

Circles with Rhythm and Space

Create two circles, one inside the other. The one on the outside will be larger. The inside circle will walk to the right and the outside circle will walk to the left.

Both circles will create a similar rhythm as you walk. Allow the same space between all the walkers.

The task is for the ones in the inner circle to rhythmically move into the outer circle one at a time and the others to readjust keeping the same distance between each other.

Now let's reverse this and those in the outer circle may change to the inner circle, one at a time, always adjusting the spaces so they stay the same.

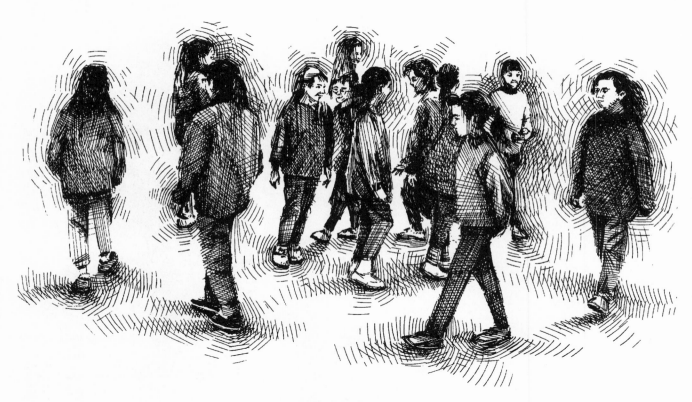

Variations

Try other types of locomotion such as skipping, running or jumping. How about trying different types of rhythms?

Art

Using a compass make lots of circles and let them intertwine with each other. You may want to color the spaces and shapes created.

Using different sizes and colored circles, let's create a circle picture. We can make a new design or something familiar.

Using sponges shaped in a circle, let's create sponge circle paintings.

CLOCKS

Types of Clocks

Can you think of different clocks?
There is the cuckoo clock,
the grandfather clock,
the kitchen clock,
the alarm clock,
the wrist watch,
What else?
The digital clock,
pocket watch.

Individual Clocks

Today we will be clocks telling time.

Decide what type of clock you will be. While we are looking at our large clock, use your arms to show us twelve o'clock. Yes, both arms are reaching straight over your head.

How about three o'clock? Good! Your left arm is the minute hand, stretching over your head, while your right arm is the hour hand, stretched straight to your right side.

Have a large clock in front of you.

Now *you* choose a time for us to guess. If we are right you can make a sound for each number. For example if you are a cuckoo clock that says five o'clock, you can say cuckoo five times.

If you are a grandfather clock you can make deep bongs five times and so forth. You decide what kind of sounds you want to make.

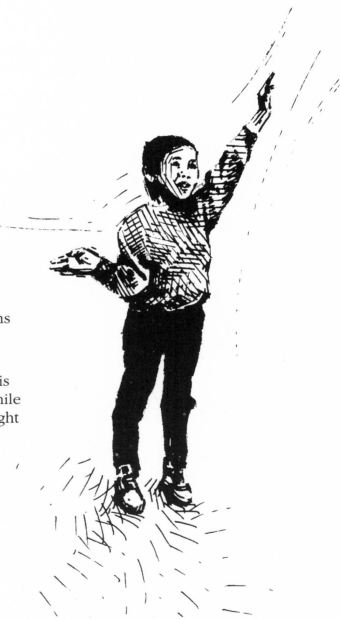

Group Clock

Make a circle with yarn on the floor, large enough for twelve children to sit around.

Twelve children can take the places of the numerals on the clock. Two more children will be the hands of the clock. Sheila, you may call out the time.

The two who are the hour and minute hands can adjust their bodies to point to the time called out. The numbers for that time may stand up and jump or make some other movement to indicate the time. Another way is for one child to use her legs as the hour and minute hands.

The twelve children around the clock may also find different ways of expressing the numbers or creating the circle.

You may all choose to tap the floor with your hands or stamp with your feet the appropriate number of beats when a new time is called out.

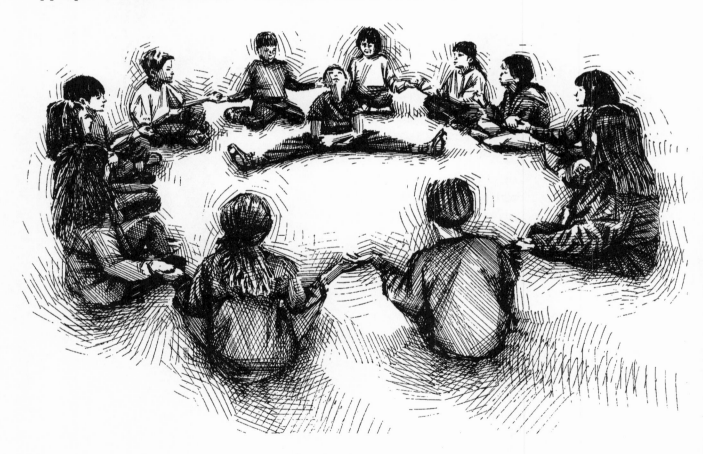

Discussion

What is your favorite time of day?

Tell us why.

What Time Is It?

Anita can be *it*. You will give us a time to do something. First tell us whether you are morning or afternoon. If the hands of your clock say twelve o'clock noon, the rest of us will act out what we think we should be doing at that time, such as eating. If your clock says twelve o'clock midnight, we will all show you sleeping. We will try to give everyone a turn at being the clock and acting out what is happening.

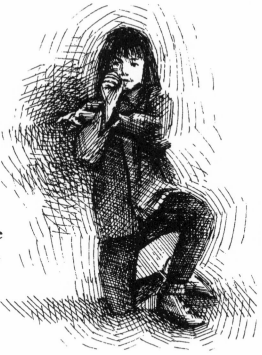

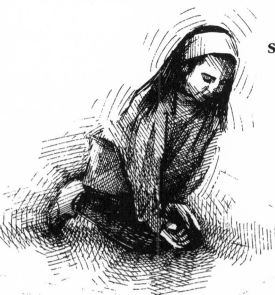

Some responses were

swinging on a swing
running a race
playing Monopoly
watching T.V.
touchdown
eating lunch
karate school
math time

Your Favorite Time of Day

Draw your favorite time of day and what you
do at that time.

Is it play time, sleeping time, vacation time
or school time?

Whatever you choose will be right for
you at this time.

What is the name of your picture?

Fast or Slow

Give us an example of time passing s l o w l y .
When you are watching the clock.

Give us an example of time moving *fast*.
When your parent calls you in from playing.
It seems that you were with your friends for
only a short time.

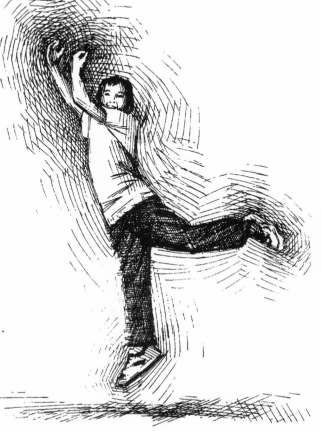

Rhythm Band

Using rhythm instruments, we will create the tick-tock music of clocks.
You can choose
rhythm sticks
bells
triangles
blocks
or other rhythm instruments.

One person can start, and the others will come in one at a time. Stop when you feel like it and then come in again.

We will make the rhythms of a clock.

You can decide as a group whether time is moving fast or slowly.

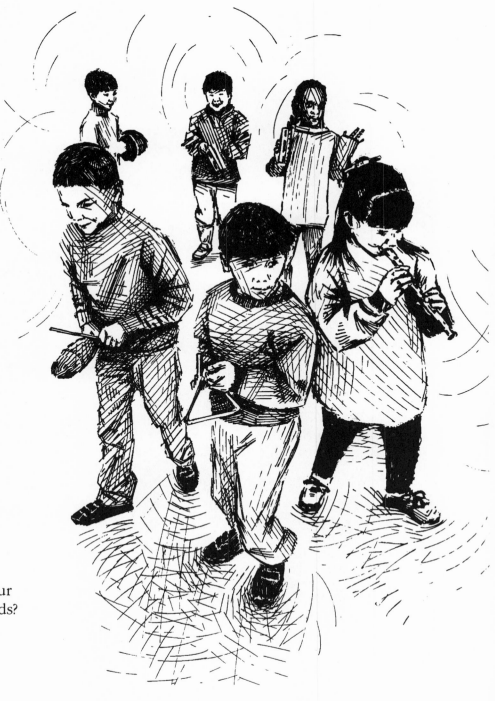

Body Sounds

Let's do the same with body sounds.

We could make clicking sounds with our mouths.

Clap our hands or stamp our feet.

How else can you use your body to make clock sounds?

ANIMALS

Can you move as these animals?

Cats
    Climb, leap, stretch, stalk, pounce, slink, curl up, slurp

Dogs
    beg, scratch, fetch, roll, dig, run

Fish
    swim, jump, leap, dive

Bees
    fly, dive, buzz, sting

Chicks
    peck, scratch, hop, waddle

Birds
    fly, soar, perch, hop

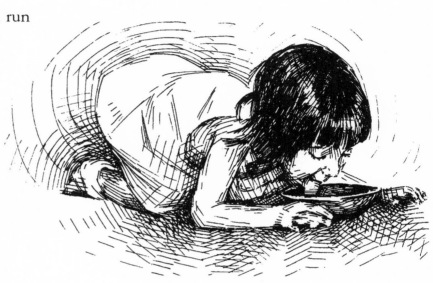

Squirrel
    run, leap, twirl, jump

Pigs
    dig, walk, wallow

Horses
    run, trot, leap, gallop

Seals
    dive, swim, balance, waddle

Snakes
    wiggle, glide, slither, slide

Bears
    climb, run, sleep, lumber

Giraffes
    stretch

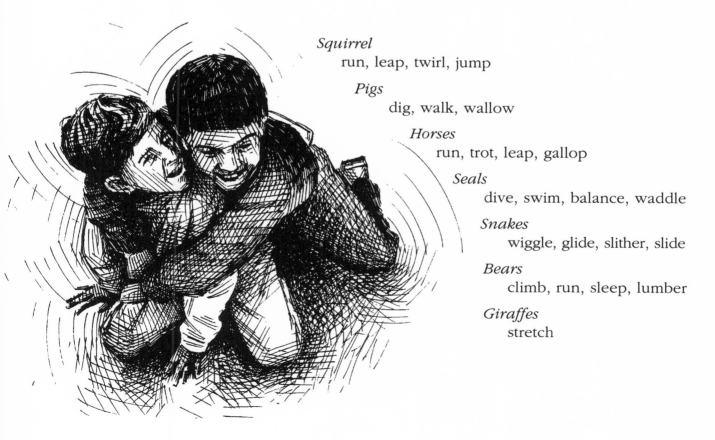

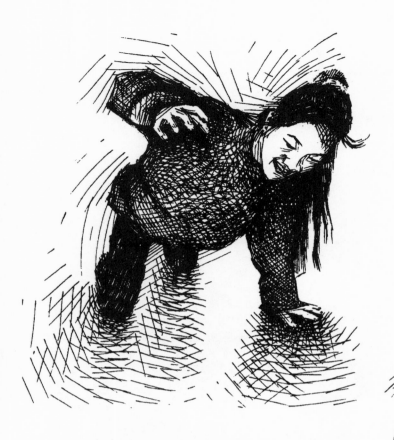

What other descriptive movement words can you add?

Macaw Parrots

How about a little story about a macaw parrot such as?

I come from deep within the Amazon jungle. I am all color and beauty. I fly gracefully through the skies and perch high above the ground in the treetops far away from humans and other predators.

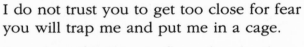

I do not trust you to get too close for fear you will trap me and put me in a cage.

I need my freedom to fly and make the world beautiful.

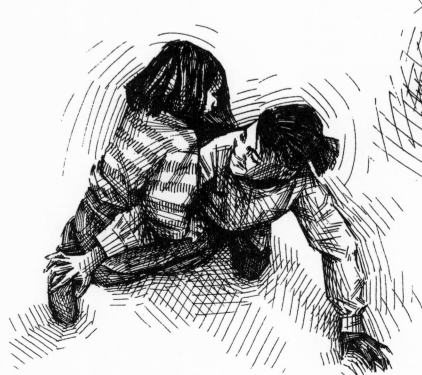

Suggested Art Materials and Equipment for the Expressive Classroom

finger paints
tempera paints
finger paint paper
tissue paper
paint brushes
clay and clay boards
masking tape
school paste
magazines
variety of collage materials
stapler
mirror
video camera

markers
oil pastels
construction paper
crepe paper
sponges
popsicle sticks
white glue
yarn
styrofoam balls
hole punch
music audiocassettes
videocassettes

water colors
chalk pastels
water color paper
newsprint pads
containers
scissors
glue sticks
buttons
streamers
floor protector
push pins
audiocassette player
tripod

Props

pillows, stuffed animals, rhythm instruments, balloons, hula hoops, soap bubbles, confetti, masks, hats and costumes, stretch fabrics, scarves, jump ropes, elastic ropes, bamboo poles, blocks of different sizes, parachutes, and a variety of balls.

Creating an Artistic Environment

Your place will be one for children and adults to be creative, intuitive, play, have fun and explore fantasy. Art materials need to be in sight and available. Don't hesitate to draw upon your art materials and equipment spontaneously when indicated.

Music

Always use music that you yourself enjoy. Have a variety of selections handy:
Music to relax to or background for guided imagery
Primal drum music that excites and energizes
Inspirational melodic music from films or the classics
Music that has a variety of rhythms to stimulate different movement
Music that different populations would relate to such as some oldies for the elderly.

Appendix A

MOVEMENT FOR THE OLDER ADULT

Dedicated to the memory of my mother, Paula Herzman

During the years I visited my mother in a nursing home, I got to know many of the other residents. I would tell them about my mother, who, as a child, would dance in the streets to the tune played by the organ grinder. On some occasions I would spontaneously dance when the nursing home residents had music sessions. Eventually I would coax some of the other residents to dance with me. They would share their pleasure with me, saying how much better they felt after dancing. With increasing frequency, I used improvisation to allow both those who were mobile as well as those in wheel chairs to experience creative movement. Most important to me, my mother smiled a lot, enjoyed herself and helped me to heal the loss of the person she had been.

After my mother died I continued the dancing experience in her honor. People who rarely got up would dance with me. Individuals who spent much of their time staring blankly into space re-energized and became more involved in socializing. I also coaxed some of the nurses, aides and other adult children who were visiting to get up and dance with their parents and other residents.

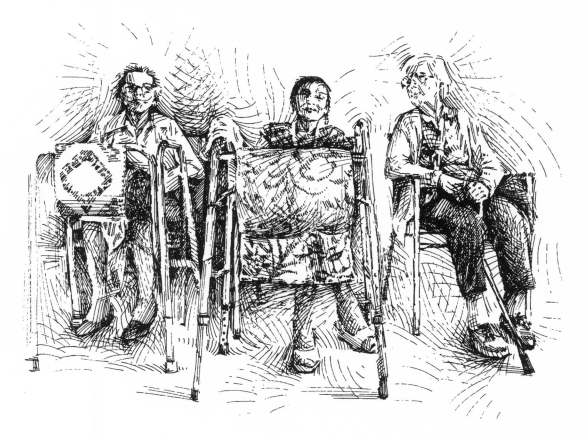

I sometimes used colorful scarves that I dramatically threw up in the air to float down on different participants. What happened was mostly spontaneous. The music I used was from the past to which the residents related. I remember hearing these songs sung by my father, Eugene L. Herzman, long ago.

Many of the movement experiences written here can be adapted for the elderly. For example, mirroring is something that all ages can enjoy. One spring I choreographed a May Pole dance, a march, a circle dance and a wheelchair dance for some of the residents and staff. It was well received by all and at the end many of the residents, visitors and staff took us up on our invitation to join in a free movement experience.

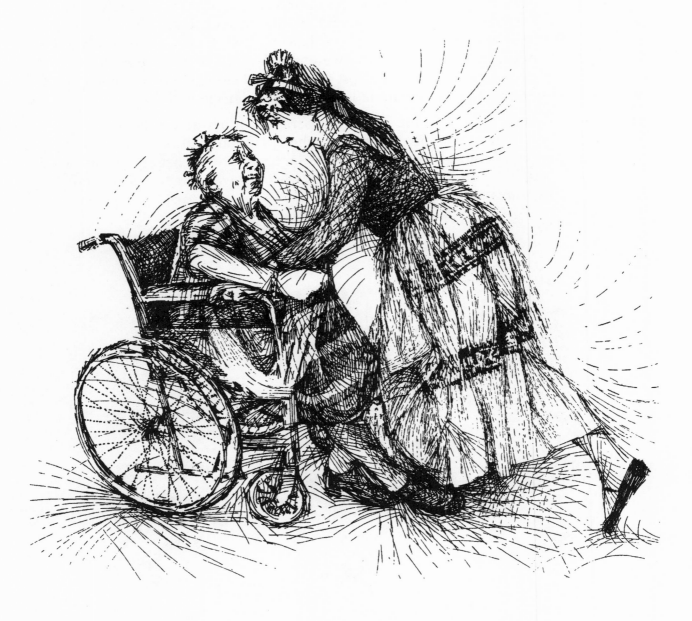

Life is movement and movement stimulates life. For the elderly, particularly those in nursing homes, it enhances self-esteem, self-worth and enables them to open up to new possibilities by stretching boundaries and increasing mobility.

Movement helps reinforce the positive by finding ways those with limits *can* move and helps them redefine themselves.

Dance becomes a way of saying yes! Yes to feelings, Yes to our bodies,
    Yes to each other,
        Yes to ourselves,
            Yes to our spaces,
                Yes to our thoughts and
                    Yes to the expressive parts of ourselves.

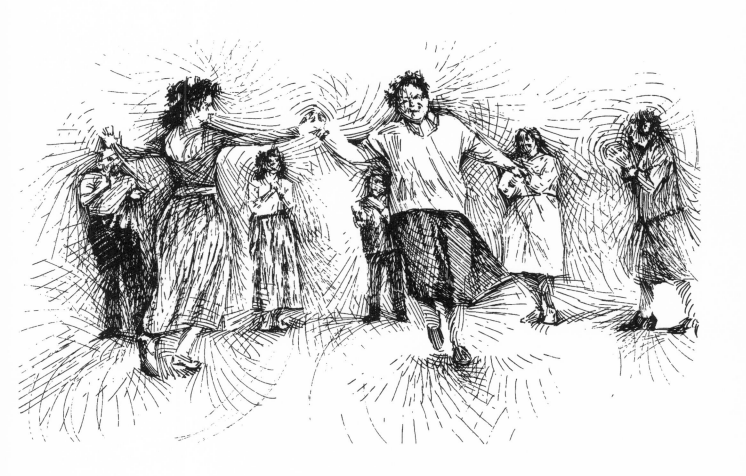

In the nursing home many of the residents shared their thoughts about their lives and feelings of being less than what they had been.

They were no longer able to take care of themselves and were sitting in chairs, looking out windows, deep in thought:

thoughts of the past, times when they were more mobile and had more control over their bodies;
    times when their lives were full of busy events,
        of being in their own homes with their own belongings,
           of being with their families,
              with their loved ones,
                watching and caring for their children,
                watching them grow,
                    watching them laugh,
                    giving and receiving love
                    and being productive
                    in the world.

        "Oh, to move again like I used to."
          "Remember how I used to dance?"

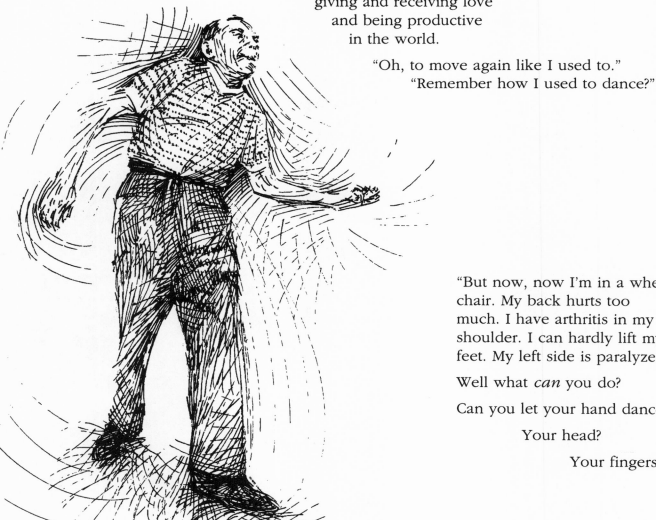

"But now, now I'm in a wheel-chair. My back hurts too much. I have arthritis in my shoulder. I can hardly lift my feet. My left side is paralyzed."

Well what *can* you do?

Can you let your hand dance?

    Your head?

        Your fingers?

Look at that wonderful hand and head dance, rekindling the spark of life that dance brings to us.

Feel the adrenalin flow,
    bringing life back into our tired bodies,
        experiencing the joy of life here and now.

Our movement is honest in that it comes from us and belongs to us. It is a reflection of how we feel, think and act.

A movement that is a walk, through intention can become a dance.

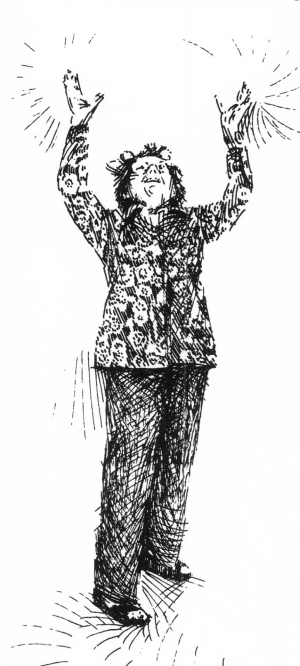

Movement can ease some of the stiffness in joints. It can ease tensions and free mobility. Movement can be healing.

What is possible? How and how much can we move?

It is important to redefine what is possible and perhaps stretch our limitations and remove the stereotypes that are limiting our vision.

The movement specialist can inspire or limit students by her expectations or lack of them. We may unnecessarily limit the older adult we care for. We must understand that dynamics and possibilities can change. Remaining unchanged and fixing our expectations limit possibilities.

Music and sound are crucial. Finding music elders can relate to is an important part of stimulating movement, life and excitement and energizing the body.

Older people are not necessarily helpless, even if in a wheelchair or in a nursing home. We need to find out and respect what is possible and then work to extend it.

Ongoing support, respect, friendship and just being there can stimulate older adults to want to extend their movement possibilities.

Many of the experiences shown here for children can also be used for adults and older adults with or without physical, emotional or mental limitations. It has more to do with attitude than with specific movements.

Some reactions of older adults to movement experiences have been

I enjoyed it.
It made me feel I was having fun.
I had a good time.
I used to be a very good dancer.
I enjoy dancing.
I always had a nice man to dance with.
It made me feel happy.
I love to dance.
I enjoy being with a good dancer.
It makes me feel that spring has sprung.
It makes me feel so gay.
It makes me feel oo la la.
Every time I dance I feel good.
I remember dancing when I was young
and I still can dance.
I would like to dance more often.

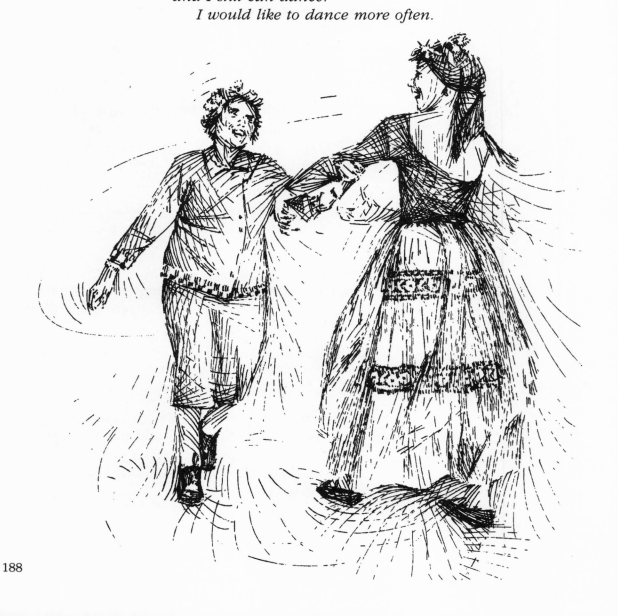

In the nursing home, the residents' participation had a positive effect on morale. They live in a closed environment and being able to break out is worthwhile. I saw looks of ecstasy on the faces of those in wheelchairs. They bent to the music to the right and left and limbered up. One woman said, "I was moving really nice to the rhythm of the music. I didn't know I could really do it. In the old days there were a lot of dance halls."

Mr. B said: "We used to go to dances pretty regularly. I had a feeling of exhilaration. It has a joyous effect and I forget everything else. It clears my mind out. Exercising my legs makes them feel better. I could walk without the stick. Makes me feel young again."

Regina in a wheelchair said: "I would rather be on my feet dancing. While I was doing it I was happy. I felt the excitement and I would do it again."

Mr. M said: "It was refreshing and enjoyable. I did the cane hop. Music will even curb a wild lion. It's a good idea for the residents to join in to be in show business. You throw yourself into it with all your energy and you forget."

Mr. H said, "It was beautiful. I used to teach dancing."

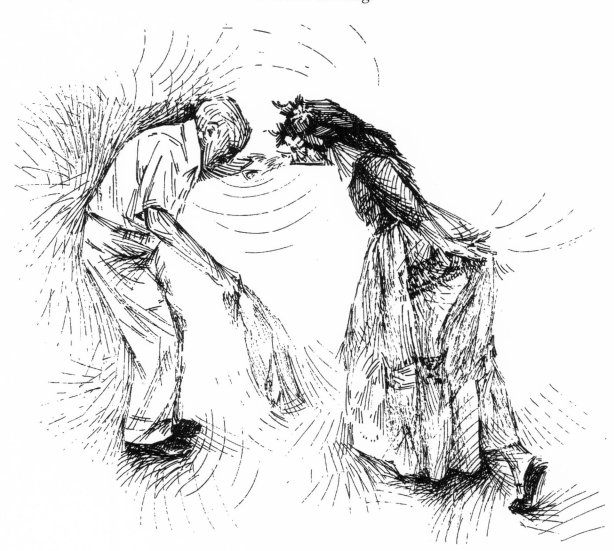

Image of Older Adults

Grandma, warmth, forgiveness, love, delicious homemade pies and cakes, presents, comfort, magic.

Retirement from life

Society fearing death cannot look in the faces of people who remind them of their inevitable destiny. Some elderly experience extreme isolation.

Movement enables communication through nonverbal means. One woman was a part of the group only through physical proximity. People need not always be actively involved to feel a part of the group.

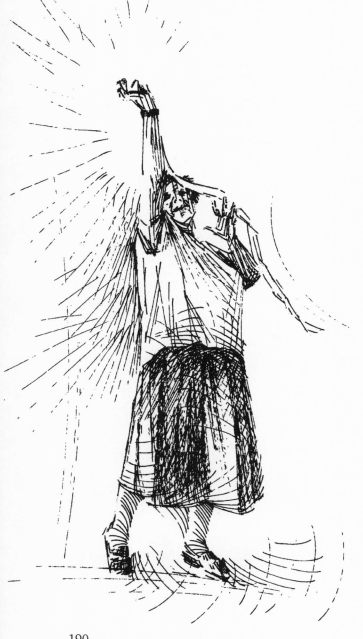

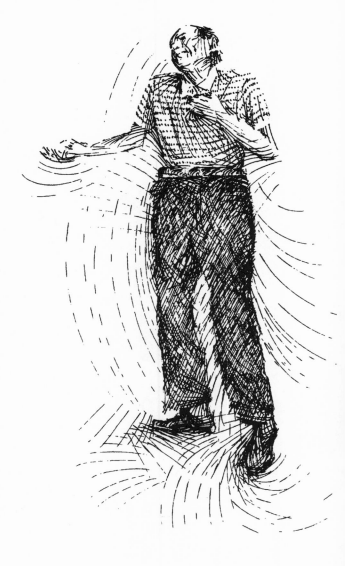

Appendix B

MOVEMENT SPECIALIST IN A PRESCHOOL MULTIHANDICAPPED CLASSROOM

Introduction

The following movement ideas came from my experiences as a movement consultant to Louise Kelsey in her multiply handicapped classroom of children ages three to five. The morning class was more developmentally delayed than the afternoon class. Because many of these children had limited communication skills, movement was able to enhance their abilities and expand their skills to relate with each other and to understand some basic concepts in education.

To a greater or lesser degree all of us are limited by our bodies, which may be perceived as imperfect. However, I feel that inside every one of us, we are perfect. It is that perfection we endeavor to reach and connect to.

After learning all of the fundamentals of movement and the foundations and theoretical bases of special education, we need to work from our heart and from a place of deep reverence and respect for all living things. When we work with children kinesthetically and through all the senses, regardless of ability, we feel and hope we will eventually reach the child and make a connection. We never know how much work or how many different ways it will take to begin communication. We never give up. It's that first spark of recognition, that first response that greatly rewards us for all our efforts. Those of us who have chosen to care for and nurture life as our life's work are privileged and have much courage.

We may not know what someone's potential is, what might spark some kind of response within a child or what is going on in a child's tremendously complicated brain. We must keep trying to reach the child in as many ways as possible. Although we sometimes get no response, we must feel and hope that at some point we will connect with them.

Being with these children, for me, is like being in a world of slow motion. My senses have more time to feel, see, touch, hear and be. I feel awed by this special environment. In the outside world we are forging ahead. We have our goals and dreams for which to strive.

In the special needs environment we cannot impose our energies, rhythm or lifestyle on these children. We enter a new dimension of time. In order to have communication we must enter and explore their special worlds by trying to hear, see, touch and feel their experience. It's the only way to reach and to be accepted by them. I had to give up my own time schedules and enter the world of a slowly unfolding flower, each petal, each emerging realm more beautiful than the last.

Pass the Yarn Ball

I place a bright red ball of yarn in my young student's hands and hold her hands on the ball with mine. Some rhythmic music is playing on the tape recorder—Scott Joplin, "The Sting." We pass the ball on to the next child, who receives it with the help of her teacher. The ball gets passed around in this manner with rhythmic counting.

    1, 2 . . . 1, 2 . . . 1, 2.

Three of the children begin to count rhythmically. Some begin to follow the ball with their eyes as it gets passed from child to child. One reaches for the ball as it gets to him (a first-time response for this child). As the movement continues the children get more and more into the rhythm: they initiate passing the ball with less help from the teacher.

Making Contact

Sometimes it feels as if we are not making any headway in establishing contact with a child. Then unexpectedly, we find we have progressed. For example, we physically moved Joyce through all the activities without getting any response from her. Joyce was sitting between my legs with my arms around her. I held Joyce's hands as I took a ball from one child and passed it on to the next. I let my hand and arms drop to my sides. Joyce picked up my hand with hers and placed it in her lap. Contact! Nonverbal communication! I was thrilled to comply.

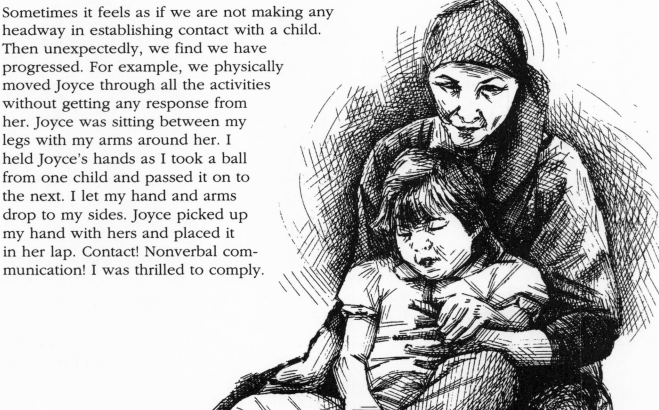

Extending the Lesson

The afternoon class has eight children. The four teachers sit between the children. After going through the previous lesson we decide to give every child a ball.

We move the ball up and down in our hands, still working rhythmically with the music. Then side to side. We tap our head with the ball saying "head" each time we tap. We then tap our stomach with the ball, saying "stomach, stomach, stomach," and so on. We proceed to combinations such as head-stomach, head-stomach, head-stomach; left shoulder-right shoulder, left shoulder-right shoulder.

In going from shoulder to shoulder we are crossing the midline, connecting left and right brain hemispheres.

What other part shall we tap with the ball? Knees. Let's cross our legs in front and go from knee to knee.

When we moved the ball from side to side, holding it in both hands, one little boy rhythmically placed the ball in one hand and then the other. Back and forth, back and forth. Look what Randy is doing. Let's all try to do that, going from one hand to the other.

When I observe a child trying something on his own, I give positive reinforcement by acknowledging the behavior and adding it to our lesson.

The children then have a chance to place the ball in the bag, saying "in."

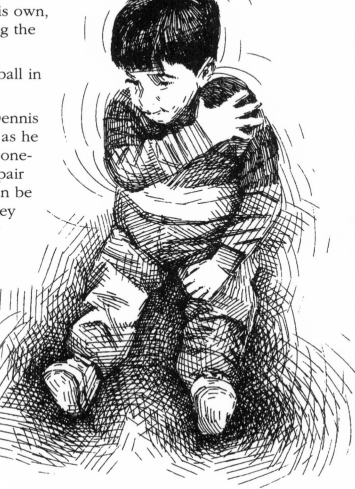

Some time after our group yarn ball activity, Dennis went to get the yarn balls on his own as soon as he heard the music and began to count one-two, one-two in rhythm. He had just recently begun to pair verbal language and signing. Aural memory can be especially strong with these children. When they hear music, they spontaneously do the activity they have come to associate with it.

Dennis is becoming a more independent and self-motivated learner in hearing the stimulus from music instead of solely from the teacher. He initiated purposeful activity for the first time and entertained himself with something meaningful. Music and props seem to be a powerful stimulus for all the children, eliciting growth and responsiveness.

Mirroring

We all sat in a circle. Many of these children were considered autistic. One little boy was engrossed with the movement of his hands and fingers.

Let's all move our hands like Danny.

The teachers helped the rest of the children move their hands. Another little girl consistently manipulated her ear. She was very sensitive to sound.

Let's all move our ear like Alice.

Alice smiled at our joining in on what she considered her movement. We continued this way for all the children.

First we asked for a movement and when one was not forthcoming we picked up on a movement the child was doing naturally or was doing for self-stimulation.

In these instances it gave the teacher the opportunity to move into the child's world, to acknowledge the children's movements, create an environment of group acceptance and make it more meaningful for all.

Often these self-stimulating movements were expanded by making them larger or smaller. We were thus able to increase the child's movement vocabulary. What began as an isolated, self-stimulating movement developed into a purposeful and meaningful activity.

The children with heightened awareness enjoyed taking leadership. Everyone followed their movements.

Even some of our children with very limited movement ability felt important in the role of leader. No matter how small or limited the movement, the rest of the class was able, in some way, to imitate it.

Face and Head Awareness

Gently touch your face.

My three-year-old partner, Mary, with
Down's syndrome, keeps her hands in
a fist.

I gently open them and place them on her
face, helping her caress her own cheeks.

She smiles.
    Now your nose.
        Say "nose" as she touches her nose.
        Eyes. Say "eyes." "Mouth."

My partner also wants to touch my eyes,
nose, cheeks, ears as we name them.
I let her, sometimes reopening her hand.
I gently caress her face at the same time.
She is delighted and goes back and forth
to her face and then to mine.

Now your neck, hair.
    Be gentle.
        Touch gently.

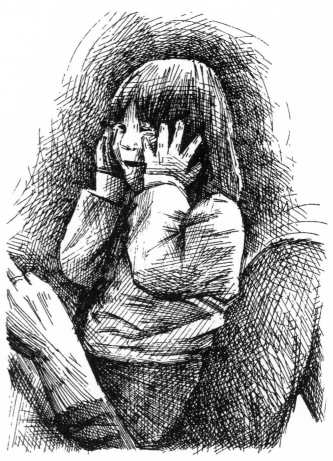

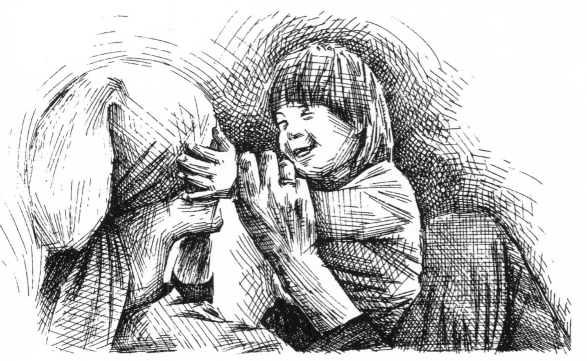

My touch shows that she can feel a gentle touch as well as hear the word. She loses interest in my face and head, looks around and then reaches out toward another child. Her touch is more of a smack than a touch. I place my hands over hers and together we explore the other child gently.

Gently feel the nose, cheeks.

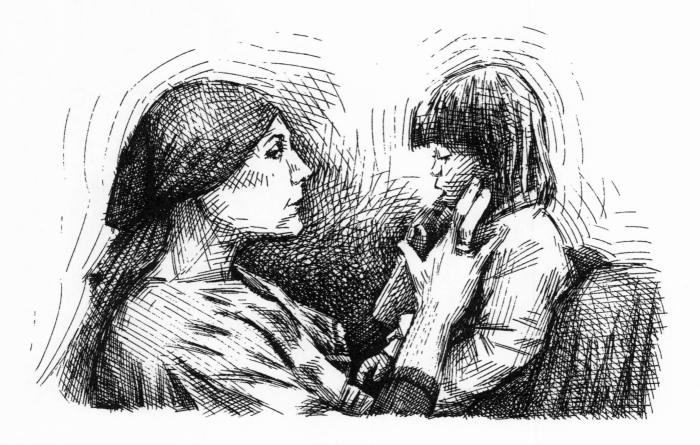

I also encourage Mary's new partner, Joseph, to explore Mary. They smile as they become engrossed in each other's face and head, as a new way of experiencing touch. Mary had often been touched harshly. We go on to touching the back, shoulders, arms, hands, fingers and feet.

We love our bodies.

We are kind to our bodies.

Touch can feel nice.

We can make our friends feel nice by touching them gently.

Some children like to have their shirts taken off. The touch feels good on their skin, arms, back, chest. One child continues to remove shoes and socks. We accommodate by stroking his feet and counting his toes. He smiles.

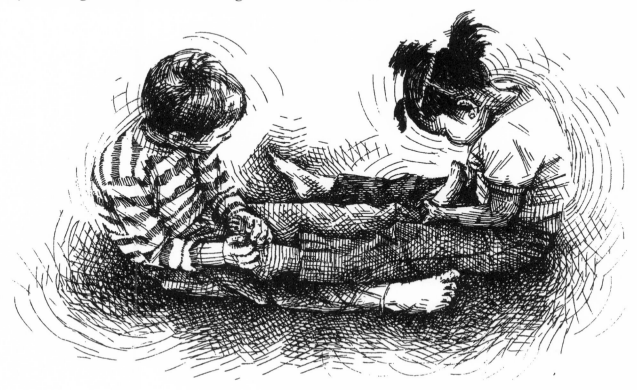

Touch

Touch is a very important part of our work. Some children do not like to touch or be touched. Other children always want to touch and then we have the challenge of teaching appropriate touching. For a child who doesn't like to be touched we never force it. Sometimes a child will work with an adult rather than a peer or with a peer rather than an adult. Sometimes a child will work only with a particular partner. Self-touching can help decrease tactile defensiveness.

After working daily for a few weeks we notice a decided improvement in one low-functioning child. His usual behavior of grabbing, scratching others and pulling hair changes to become more gentle toward the other children.

Children can be helped to become more aware of themselves and how their touch affects others through constant feedback and different positive touching experiences. For children who have experienced harsh touch, gentle touching can particularly be an important learning experience.

A scarf or rope may be used as a medium between two children who cannot tolerate direct contact. The rope can be a way of helping children connect while honoring their need for no contact. Making the rope shorter and shorter can eventually desensitize the children.

Tubular Fabric

I sat inside a large, stretchy bag with four-year-old Brian, who developmentally was about six months old. We faced each other. He was smiling. He liked being contained with me. The fabric hugging his back helped give Brian support so that it was easier for him to sit up. He would usually collapse, with his head down to the floor. I said "up" and raised my arms up. Brian followed my hands with his eyes.

"You put *your* hands up."

I took his hands in mine, raising them. "Good Brian! Up!" Brian looked up at our hands gleefully. "Now down" and I brought our hands down. I repeated that numerous times, smiling into Brian's face. I let go of his hands. "Now you do it, Brian. Up," and I brought my hands up. Brian raised his hands.

"You're doing it!" Brian raised his own hands when I said up. Brian was grinning broadly. He knew he'd done something wonderful.

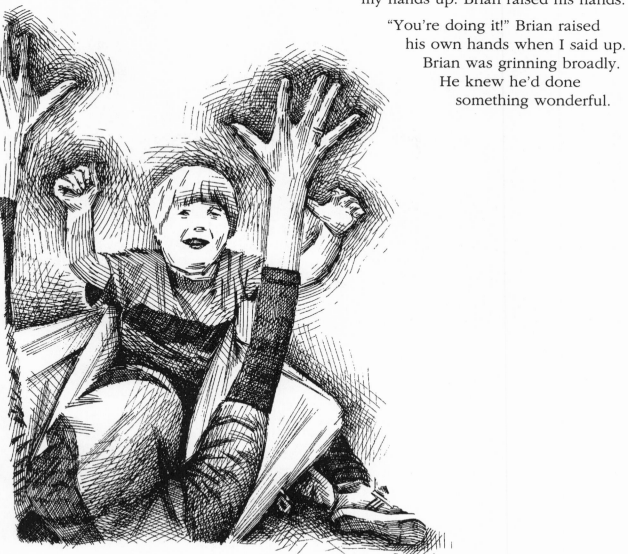

We stayed together inside the fabric tube for half an hour, moving and communicating in different ways. We swung our arms, clapped our hands, held hands and moved our arms all around to the music. We expanded our movement to include our upper bodies. Pushed, pulled, up and down. Brian moved with me, maintaining eye contact throughout. He stayed focused and thoroughly enjoyed himself.

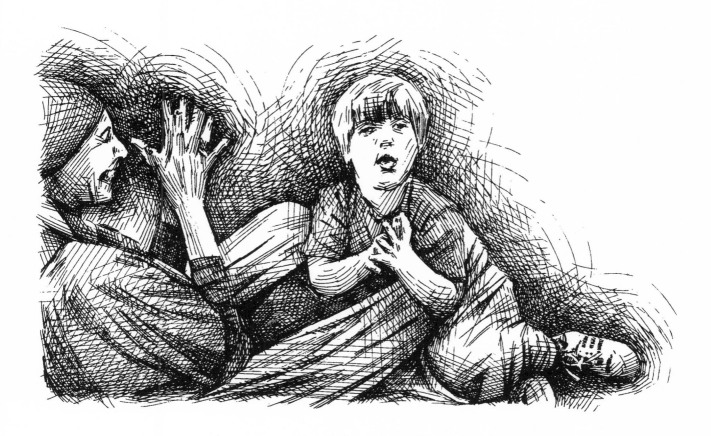

The stretch fabric gave us a boundary that defined a mutual space for us to share together and gave Brian physical support. When we moved back in the jersey sack, tension helped us move forward again. It supported Brian, socially allowing him to be responsive to me, the enclosure, and our involvement.

The more we were together, the more Brian tuned in to my voice and body movement. This little boy was fully participating rather than just reacting. There was true social interaction as he responded to my raised arms by lifting his arms up, keeping eye contact, tracking our movements and smiling the entire time.

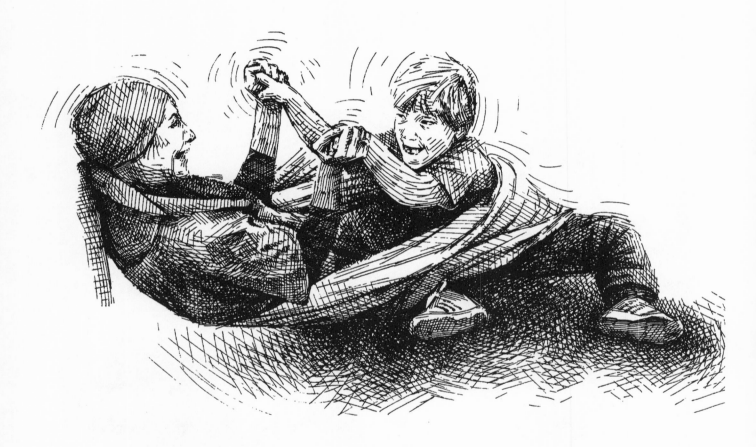

At a moment of rest, Brian reached out to me with his hands, nonverbally communicating that he wanted more movement. I obliged.

Brian also began to initiate his own movements. He clapped his hands and I followed him. Then he shook his hand and I followed, shaking mine. Sometimes we had been able to get Brian to imitate our movement, but this time he initiated his own movements.

When I returned to Brian's class two weeks later, Brian reached out for my hands. Another first. Brian's connection to another person, a connection beyond himself to the outside world had been made.

Appendix C

MOVEMENT WORKSHOP TO SUMMARIZE A BRAINSTORMING WEEKEND

In the summer of 1990, a group of us from all areas of education came together to share our visions, expressed in words such as *holistic, global, ecological, future oriented* and *progressive, encouraging diversity, cooperation* and *creativity.* The purpose was to form a coalition of people from different movements and perspectives who hold a unifying vision. On the last day I brought the group together in a movement experience to share the results of personal and group efforts.

Individual Movement

Music: *Transfer Blue*

Create your vision of "whole" as it has been evolving for you these last three days. It may not be totally formed; still you can let the ideas and feelings shape themselves into your body and take form.

Partners—Mirroring

Music: *Silk Road Suite*

Find one other person and create a language to shape your ideas, thoughts and feelings. Decide nonverbally who will lead and who will mirror.

Groups of Four—Sculpting

Music: *Star Wars*

Each of you may take turns creating your vision of holistic education by sculpting your image with your three partners. Then place yourself into the image. What is your role in what you have created? You will have a minute to orally share that image with each other.

Groups of Eight—Levels

(See *A Moving Experience*)

Music: Pas de Deux from the *Nutcracker Suite*

While giving the instructions to create the levels movement activity, the author will be saying: We all have our individual ideas. Sometimes they fit with others and sometimes we stand alone. We operate on many different levels. We will manifest this. Sometimes we have to begin at the bottom, and sometimes our images, ideas, feelings get actualized at the top or anywhere in between. We all have our own vision. We are all creating beautiful visions and we will take a moment to appreciate each other.

PROFESSIONAL ORGANIZATIONS

American Art Therapy Association
1202 Allanson Road
Mundelein IL 60060
(708) 949-6064

American Association for Music Therapy
PO Box 27177
Philadelphia, PA 19118
(215) 242-4450

American Dance Guild
31 West 21st Street, 3rd Floor
New York, NY 10010

American Dance Therapy Association
2000 Century Plaza, Suite 108
Columbia, MD 21044
(410) 997-4040

American Society of Group Psychotherapy and Psychodrama
6728 Old McLean Village Drive
McLean VA 22101
(703) 556-9222

Association for Childhood Education International
11501 Georgia Avenue, Suite 315
Wheaton, MD 20902
1-800-423-3563

Association for Supervision and Curriculum Development
1250 North Pitt Street
Alexandria, VA 22314-1453
(703) 549-9110

Dance and the Child International
USA Representative, daCi
293 RB Brigham Young University
Provo, UT 84602
(801) 378-5086

International Arts Medicine Association
3600 Market Street
Philadelphia, PA 19104

Kennedy Center Alliance for Arts Education Network
The Education Department
The Kennedy Center
Washington, DC 20566-0001

National Association for the Education of the Young Child (NAEYC)
1834 Connecticut Avenue, NW
Washington, DC 20009-5786
1-800-424-2460

National Dance Association (NDA): American Alliance for Health,
Physical Education, Recreation and Dance (AAPHERD)
1900 Association Drive
Reston, VA 22091

National Association for Drama Therapy
19 Edwards Street
New Haven, CT 06511

National Association for Poetry Therapy
225 Williams Street
Huron, OH 44839

Organisation Mondiale Pour L'Education Prescolaire (OMEP)
World Organization for Early Childhood Education
U.S. National Committee
733 Amsterdam Avenue, 22 E
New York, NY 10025

SUGGESTED READINGS

Bagley, Michael, and Karin Hess. 1982. *200 Ways of Using Imagery in the Classroom*. Woodcliff, N.J.: New Dimensions of the 80s. (P.O. Box 8559, Woodcliff, NJ 07675.)

A guide for developing imagination and creativity in elementary students.

Benzwie, Teresa. 1987. *A Moving Experience: Dance for Lovers of Children and the Child Within*. Tucson, Ariz.: Zephyr Press.

Integrates curriculum areas with movement and self-esteem.

Cherry, Clair. 1981. *Think of Something Quiet: A Guide for Achieving Serenity n Early Childhood Classrooms*. Belmont, Calif.: Pitman Learning.

Chemfeld, Mimi Brodsky. 1983. *Creative Activities for Young Children*. New York: Harcourt Brace Jovanovich.

This book is packed with hundreds of ideas for children to experience life lovingly and creatively.

Chime Time Catalogue

Anyone who wishes to order the parachute, Body Sox, Co-Oper Band and other such materials may call 1-800-477-5075, or write 1 Sportime Way, Atlanta, GA, 30340.

Cohen, Bonnie Bainbridge. *Sensing, Feeling, and Action: The Experiential Anatomy of Body Mind Centering*.

Contact Quarterly Dance Journal, 1980–1992. (P.O. Box 603, Northampton, MA 01061, 413-586-1181.)

Dance as Education.

This publication, a pictorial essay on dance as curricula, is the result of a conference held October 22–25, 1976, at the John F. Kennedy Center for the Performing Arts, Washington, D.C., as part of a National Dance Association Project on Issues and Concerns in Dance education. You can get a copy from AAHPERD Promotion Unit, 1201 Sixteenth St NW, Washington, DC 20036.

Educators for Social Responsibility. 1983. *Perspectives: A Teaching Guide to Concepts of Peace*. Cambridge, Mass.: Educators for Social Responsibility. (11 Garden St., Cambridge, MS 02138, 617-492-1764.)

Many activities to foster world and personal peace and self-esteem.

Fanck, Frederick. 1979. *The Awakened Eye*. New York: Random House, Vintage.

This book is a companion volume to *The Zen of Seeing*. It offers a meditative way of seeing, being, and drawing.

Fraser, Diane Lynch. 1991. *Playdancing*. Princeton Book Co.

This book is about developing creativity in young children and helping them discover it.

Gawain, Shakti. 1979. *Creative Visualization.* New York: Bantam.

> The philosophy of fulfillment through mental energy and affirmations. Many exercises and guided meditations.

Gilbert, Anne Green. 1992. *Creative Dance for All Ages.* Reston, Va.: National Dance Association, an association of the American Alliance for Health, Physical Education, Recreation and Dance. (1900 Association Drive, Reston, VA 22091.)

Hendricks, Gay, and Russell Wills. 1975. *The Centering Book: Awareness Activities for Children, Parents and Teachers.* Englewood Cliffs, N.J.: Prentice-Hall.

Jacob, Ellen. *Dancing,* rev. ed. New York: Variety Arts. (305 Riverside Dr., Suite 4 A, New York, NY 10025, 212-316-0399.)

> Has practical, specific advice and information on many aspects of dance.

Lee, Alison. *A Handbook of Creative Dance and Drama.* Portsmouth, N.H.: Heinemann Educational Books. (361 Hanover St., Portsmouth, NH 03801-3959.)

> A collection of practical ideas with the use of imagery to guide you through a drama course for young children.

Lloyd, Marcia. *Adventures in Creative Movement Activities: A Guide for Teaching.* Idaho State University: Dance and Physical Education Department. (Pocatello, ID 83209.)

Purcell, Theresa. 1994. *Teaching Children Dance: Becoming a Master Teacher.* Champaign, IL: Human Kinetics. (P.O. Box 5076, Champaign, IL 61825-5076.)

> Developmentally appropriate learning experiences in dance to incorporate in physical education programs.

Stinson, Sue. 1988. *Dance for Young Children: Finding the Magic in Movement.* National Dance Association.

> Movement experiences sensitively written for children to learn about themselves, others and their environment.

Stinson, Sue, Teresa Benzwie, Roberta Pasternack, Rae Pica, Elsa Rosey. 1990. *Guide to Creative Dance for the Young Child.* Reston, Va.: National Dance Association.

Stinson, William, ed. 1989. *Moving and Learning for the Young Child.* Presentations from the early childhood conference, "Forging the Linkage between Moving and Learning for Preschool Children," Washington, D.C., December 1–4, 1988.

Teresa Benzwie brings you more MOVEMENT experiences with...

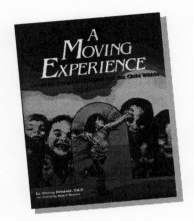

A MOVING EXPERIENCE
Dance for Lovers of Children and the Child Within
by Teresa Benzwie
Grades PreK–6

Let *A Moving Experience* dance its way into your heart, as it has for thousands of others. More than 100 exercises help children discover qualities of space, time, numbers, their bodies, and rhythm.

216 pages, 8 1/2" x 11", softbound.
1003-W . . . $29

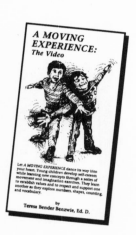

A MOVING EXPERIENCE: THE VIDEO
by Teresa Benzwie
Grades PreK–6

In this outstanding video, Benzwie guides her kindergarten students through many of the activities from the book, using motion and imagination.

30-minute VHS video and guide.
1701-W . . . $49

ORDER FORM
☎ Please include your phone number in case we have questions about your order.

Qty.	Item #	Title	Unit Price	Total
	1003-W	A Moving Experience	$29	
	1701-W	A Moving Experience: The Video	$49	

Name _____
Address _____
City _____
State _____ Zip _____
Phone (_____) _____
E-mail _____

Method of payment (check one):
❏ Check or Money Order ❏ Visa
❏ MasterCard ❏ Purchase Order Attached
Credit Card No. _____
Expires _____
Signature _____

Subtotal	
Sales Tax (AZ residents, 5%)	
S & H (10% of Subtotal-min $4.00)	
Total (U.S. Funds only)	

CANADA: add 22% for S& H and G.S.T.

100% SATISFACTION GUARANTEE

Upon receiving your order you'll have 90 days of risk-free evaluation. If you are not 100% satisfied, return your order in saleable condition within 90 days for a 100% refund of the purchase price. No questions asked!

Call, Write, or FAX for your FREE Catalog!

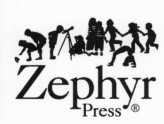

REACHING THEIR HIGHEST POTENTIAL

P.O. Box 66006-W
Tucson, AZ 85728-6006

1-800-232-2187
FAX 520-323-9402
http://www.zephyrpress.com